SURVIVING STROKE

The Story of a Neurologist and His Family

Dr. Helen Kennerley and Prof. Udo Kischka

ROBINSON

ROBINSON

First published in Great Britain in 2020 by Robinson

Copyright © Helen Kennerley and Udo Kischka, 2020

1 3 5 7 9 10 8 6 4 2

The moral right of the author has been asserted.

A CIP catalogue record for this book is available from the British Library

ISBN: 978-1-47214-446-1

Typeset in Scala by Hewer Text UK Ltd, Edinburgh
Printed and bound in Great Britain by Clays Ltd, Elcograf S.p.A.

Papers used by Robinson are from well-managed
forests and other responsible sources

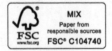

MIX
Paper from
responsible sources
FSC® C104740

Robinson
An imprint of
Little, Brown Book Group
Carmelite House
50 Victoria Embankment
London EC4Y 0DZ

An Hachette UK Company
www.hachette.co.uk

www.littlebrown.co.uk

In memory of Dr Karl Harald Kischka (1924–2019)

Contents

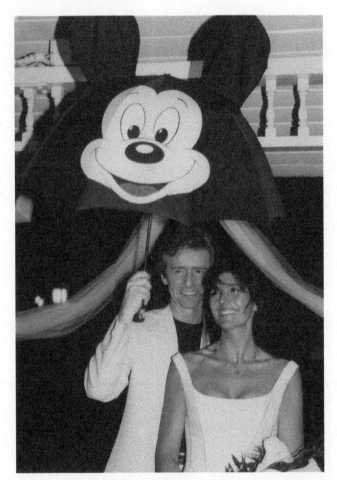

The beginning of our lives together: easier times

Preface

'This is life changing.
This is a life-changing event.'

By 2016, our life was wonderfully unremarkable. Our careers had matured, and our two children had settled into their teens. We'd had a few rough patches in the past, but things now felt on an even keel. Helen was semi-retired so that she could spend more time supporting the children and Udo was working far too hard but enjoying every minute of it. As professionals we were both doing what we wanted to do: Udo was an NHS medical consultant in a specialist neuro-rehabilitation unit in Oxford and Helen a clinical psychologist in a specialist NHS unit for cognitive behaviour therapy (CBT). Udo's skill was in helping people recover from brain injury and Helen helped people overcome psychological problems and life crises.

We knew that we were a fortunate family, as Helen tediously reminded the kids; we took none of our contentment for granted and that's one of the reasons it felt so wrong when it was snatched away overnight. Within hours of his stroke Udo uttered the words, 'This is a life-changing event, Helen.' He was right. At once our lives were radically altered and we were about to embark on a journey for which we were ill prepared. You might have thought that with Udo's specialist knowledge of stroke and Helen's training in managing emotional problems we would be uncommonly well equipped to deal with the onslaught of shocks that follow a severe brain injury, but we struggled. As individuals, as a married couple and as a family, we struggled. But we also survived. After a fashion we pulled through and a couple of years down the line we live life again. It's not the life that we expected, and it is certainly not the one that we wanted, but it's a recognisable, purposeful way of being that even has us counting our blessings from time to time.

Everyone, every family that endures a stroke, will have a unique story to tell. Some will fare better than us and some worse, but we wanted to share our tale in the hope that it might help others. Despite feeling so at sea in those early days, looking back we thought that we might have something to offer. We thought that if we put our neurologist and psychologist heads together we could produce something that might give the information, orientation and direction that would have helped us. That's not to say that we weren't given excellent care and information – we were, but we found ourselves so easily overwhelmed that we often couldn't remember our neuropsychological conversations with professionals. So, we thought that it would be helpful to have some written material explaining stroke and some tried-and-tested strategies that help people cope. That's why we kick off with a chapter from Udo called 'What Is a Stroke?' and we end the book with Helen's overview of CBT and how it might be useful when the time is right. And in between these two chapters is our family's story, simply because we found it helpful and healing when others shared their experiences with us.

As Udo was so very poorly in the early days and because the stroke continues to affect his motor and cognitive skills, Helen took the lead in writing the text with constant input from Udo and some contributions from our children, although they didn't want us to use their names – that's why you'll see 'our daughter'

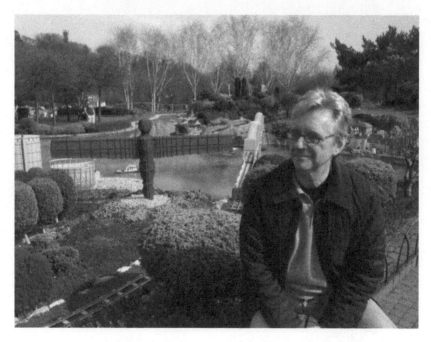

Udo's 60th birthday: a family outing to Legoland

or 'our son' in the text. It's not quite as elegant as naming them but it is what they wanted. There were heated debates over the choice of words and shared, yet conflicting, recollections of precise events, but we eventually got there. Interestingly, having a joint project that was meaningful also helped in reconciling us to a new way of being together.

Another joint project for all survivors of stroke is simply that of recovery – so often a family affair – and we hope that this text offers some help in achieving it.

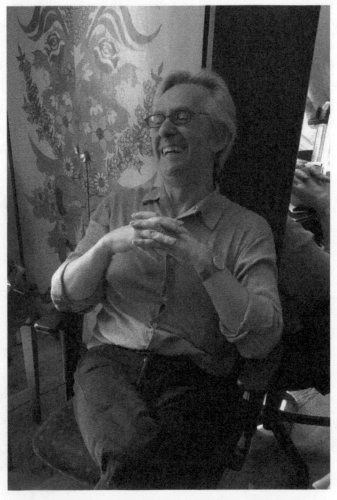

Happier times in Heidelberg just before Udo's stroke

1

What Is a Stroke? Udo Kischka

For over twenty years I had worked as a consultant in neurological rehabilitation, with people who had suffered strokes. So, it was ironic that, at the age of sixty-two, I had a stroke, a large one.

I was simply running for a train. Suddenly I felt a pain in the right side of my head and noticed a mild weakness and loss of sensation in my left arm and leg, but I was still able to climb aboard. It dawned on me that I might well have had a small bleed in my brain. However, the weakness and sensory loss on the left improved over the next hour or so and I didn't panic; in fact, I felt remarkably calm (perhaps unnaturally so). I should have left the train at the next station and called an ambulance, but my instinct was to head home instead. There I had a brief conversation with my wife, then sat at the computer in the study and worked on some reports. It was late in the evening and eventually I must have passed out, probably in the small hours of the morning, I don't remember.

I now assume that a bleed in my brain had continued to grow until I lost consciousness. My wife found me on the floor in the morning and called an ambulance. Later at the hospital, a brain CT scan showed that I had 'a large intracerebral bleed in the area of the right basal ganglia and thalamus' and I knew that our lives had changed dramatically.

Why me?

Strokes are not rare. More than 100,000 people in the UK suffer a stroke each year. That is around one stroke every few minutes in the UK. In 2016 I was one of the 100,000 and it was down to my age (stroke is considered an illness of older age), a weak spot in the wall of a blood vessel in my brain and simple bad luck.

Because the general population has become older in the last fifty years most stroke specialists predicted a steady increase in stroke numbers. Surprisingly, however, this was not the case in Oxfordshire, where I happened to practise. Here a large study showed that the frequency of stroke had slightly declined between 1990 and 2010. It is assumed that this reduction was due to increasing success by general practitioners to effectively treat their patients' risk factors for stroke, so it's worth knowing what they are:

- high blood pressure,
- high cholesterol levels,
- diabetes,
- atrial fibrillation (a heart condition).

Maybe changes in lifestyle also played a role in reducing the incidence of stroke, as people became more aware of the value of certain behaviours such as:

- not smoking,
- eating a healthy diet,
- drinking alcohol only in moderation,
- getting regular gentle workouts,
- maintaining a healthy weight,
- reducing stress.

What the study strongly suggests is that we can take steps to reduce the risk of stroke and even if, like me, you have had a stroke it is still important to try to live a healthy life so that you limit the likelihood of having another. I considered myself healthy before my stroke – I did not smoke or drink alcohol, my weight was normal, and I was reasonably fit, so I have made sure to stick to my healthy regime as I do not want to increase the chances of another brain bleed. However, I am now under much closer medical scrutiny in order to decrease the chance of a second stroke, which is as it should be. If you have had a stroke, then you too should be under a watchful medical eye from now on.

What is a stroke?

A stroke occurs when the blood supply to part of the brain is disrupted, causing damage to brain cells. It can happen to any of us. If you research famous people who've suffered stroke you see a large and diverse population including: Emilia Clarke, Tina Turner, A. A. Milne, Ronnie Biggs, all of whom survived. Some strokes are minor and don't cause much damage, but some are more severe and are literally life changing. Strokes do tend to be more common in old age as our brain vessels become narrower and harder, but they can also occur in younger people, and sadly even in children, although this is rare.

There are two types of stroke, haemorrhagic and ischaemic:

A **haemorrhagic stroke** is characterised by the bursting of a blood vessel in the brain, resulting in a bleeding into the brain. This type of stroke is often accompanied by a severe headache and weakness on one side of the body. The underlying cause of the burst is usually a weakness in the wall of a blood vessel that ruptures when the blood pressure rises, as was the case when I ran as hard as I could to catch the train. Sometimes the vulnerability in a blood vessel is caused by a **brain aneurysm** – part of an artery wall that has ballooned out and become weak. If diagnosed, this is a treatable condition and some aneurysms never cause any symptoms – but some do rupture and result in a brain bleed.

Whatever the cause, bleeding in the brain puts pressure on the surrounding tissues, damaging them and preventing them from functioning properly. Haemorrhagic strokes are the most life threatening of the two types of stroke but if we survive it then we can look forward to some recovery.

The second type of stroke, the **ischaemic stroke**, accounts for the majority of all strokes and is caused by a blood vessel getting blocked by a blood clot or a fragment of plaque. A blockage stops blood getting to the brain and this starves it of oxygen and glucose. If this happens, brain cells die in the area of the blockage. There is another condition known as a **transient ischaemic attack** (TIA) where the blood supply to the brain is only temporarily interrupted. This is often referred to as a mini-stroke and people tend to recover quite quickly. However, TIAs are frequently a warning sign for a more serious stroke so they should always be taken seriously, and emergency services should be called as early intervention is crucial.

The symptoms of stroke that you must look out for are typically:

- changes to one side of the body (the face dropping on one side and arms or legs becoming weak or numb),
- speech becoming slurred or garbled or sometimes a person cannot speak at all.

You should seek help as soon as you notice these symptoms, although, as my experience illustrates, we don't always think clearly when we are having a stroke.

Can someone recover from a stroke?

It is an alarming fact that some of us won't survive the stroke. However, those of us who do will make some recovery. In recent years it has become increasingly clear that the brain is capable of repair and repurposing. The term used to describe this is **plastic** and in the neurosciences we talk about **brain plasticity**, meaning that the brain can change and adapt even after it has been injured. This has been a really exciting finding as it means that the brain can partially regrow and form new connections. In effect, it can repair and rewire itself and importantly for stroke sufferers this means that some degree of recovery is possible both through healing of tissue and because healthy parts of the brain can take over the functions of the damaged parts. Areas of the brain that used only to perform one task can sometimes take on a different task that compensates for the damage caused by the stroke, so this also aids recovery.

The overall message here is that there is hope of some degree of recovery following a stroke. There is even more hope if we are offered rehabilitation of a high standard. Even years after a stroke, brain plasticity and recovery can be at work. In his book about his own experience of suffering a brain bleed, *My Year Off*, Robert McCrum described relearning to type using both hands twenty years after his stroke had weakened his left hand and arm.

McCrum's story of his stroke and his recovery is a moving and powerful account of what he called his 'brain attack' and there are other informative and often inspiring personal accounts of the experience of having a stroke. If you read some of these texts what you will see is that everyone's experience and recovery is slightly different, but there are some factors that consistently predict the outcome of the stroke. These are: the age of the person, the size of the stroke and where it is in the brain.

Age

Quite simply put, the younger we are when we suffer any type of brain injury, the better our outlook. A younger brain is better at repairing itself or recruiting other parts of the brain to take on new work. It would have been to my neurological advantage to have had my stroke at a younger age, but even in my seventh decade there was still much scope for recovery.

Size of stroke

Again, there is usually a relatively simple correlation: the smaller the stroke, the less damage there is and therefore the better the outlook. Some strokes are so small that people hardly notice that they have had one (or more), and they get on with life without any obvious disability. My brain bleed was classified as 'large', so we knew that recovery might be slow and limited, yet right from the start the doctors anticipated progress – and they were right to do so.

Site of the stroke

Now things get more complicated and it might be helpful to learn a few things about the brain at this point.

Although it is compact enough to sit on the palm of the hand, our brain comprises one hundred billion brain cells – that's eleven zeros. There are even more connections linking these brain cells (or neurones), enabling communication and growth, so this explains why our brains can achieve so much. Our brain keeps us alive by regulating our heartbeat, breathing and digestion. Our brain helps us to move, sit, walk and stand. It processes pain, sounds and sights, tastes and smells. It shapes our personality, generates (and controls) emotions, perceptions and thoughts – which in turn guide our behaviour. Brains hold our memories for facts, experiences and skills. They help us sleep at the right time, stay upright when we sit, resist distractions when we need to focus yet be alert to things around us. When our brain is damaged by a stroke we can lose some of these abilities.

Typically, and perhaps predictably, stroke survivors show some change in their ability to:

- control their body movements and/or
- manage thinking processes and/or
- express emotions appropriately and/or
- behave appropriately.

Some changes are minor and short lived while others might persist. I experienced changes in all these areas: I couldn't move the left side of my body, I was muddled, my concentration and memory were really bad, I was tearful, I slept much more than usual, and I had very little energy to do things. Two years on I still struggle with movement, but my thinking processes have improved, I'm less likely to be moved to tears, my sleep pattern is gradually becoming more normal and my energy and ability to initiate things is continually improving.

Brains look like a gigantic walnut with a wrinkled surface and two distinct halves: the left brain and the right brain (also called the left and right hemispheres). Oddly, the left side of the brain controls the right side of our bodies and the right side of the brain controls the left side. Thus, the motor areas in the right side of our brain move the left arm and leg, and vice versa. My stroke was in the right hemisphere close to these motor areas and as a result I couldn't move my left arm and leg and my face drooped on the left side.

The two sides of the brain have different roles. In most people the left side is specialised in processing language and detail. This means that people with a stroke in the left side of the brain often cannot understand spoken and written language or they cannot express themselves in speaking or writing. They also have a weakness in their right arm and leg.

The right side of the brain is specialised in appreciating music and art and in visualising 3-dimensional objects and orientating us in a building or a city and realising 'the big picture'. It is these abilities that are often disturbed after a right-hemisphere stroke.

We function well because of the cooperation between the two sides of our brains so fortunately the two hemispheres are connected by a thick band of nerves called the **corpus callosum**. This ensures good communication and 'teamwork'. If one side of the brain is not functioning well, our overall performance suffers. My wife asked why my right side was weak and some of my verbal abilities impaired given that I had a perfectly functioning left hemisphere. I had to explain that my undamaged left hemisphere was no longer 'perfectly functioning' now that it had lost some essential input from the right side of my brain.

Each side of the brain has specialised areas: different parts of the brain do different work. Some parts help us move, some parts store memories, some parts help decision making, for example. The diagram below shows the functions of different parts of the brain.

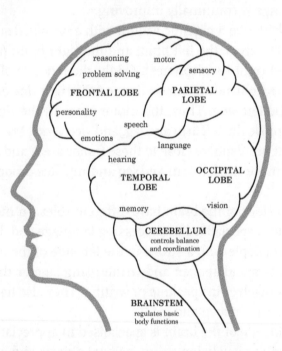

The **brainstem** connects the brain to the spinal cord and it is at the base of the skull. It's in charge of the body's most vital functions: our breathing, heartbeat, digestion, hormones and wakefulness. We can often survive damage to other parts of the brain but not serious damage to the brainstem. You might hear the phrase 'mid-line shift' when medical staff discuss the outcome of a stroke. This happens when the internal pressures in one hemisphere push the centre line of the brain over to one side. This distorts the brainstem, which means that our vital functions can suffer. I had some mid-line shift – not a great deal, but enough to have left me with some problems with breathing and sleeping.

Close to the brain stem is the **cerebellum** and this helps us coordinate our movements, making them smooth and precise. This means that we can walk without stumbling, sit without falling and lift a cup without spilling its contents.

By far the largest part of the human brain is the **cerebrum** and this comprises the left and right hemispheres. Each hemisphere is made up of four lobes:

- **The occipital lobes** are at the back of the brain and everything we see is processed here.
- **The parietal lobes** are located at the top of the brain. They process touch and pain, carry out arithmetic, focus our attention and orientate us. They also integrate information from our different senses so that when we have a cup of tea we feel its heat, smell its aroma and taste it all at the same time.
- **The temporal lobes** are located at the sides of the brain and they process sounds and make sense of them. Memories are also processed and stored here.
- **The frontal lobes** are the most sophisticated part of the human brain, just behind our foreheads. Much of our brain functions on autopilot, but frontal lobe activity is frequently conscious, which means that we are often aware that we are thinking. These lobes enable us to problem solve, plan, reason and initiate actions. Here resides our sense of self and our ability to see the world from another person's perspective. They also have a role in controlling our emotions and impulses and developing our personality. In addition, the left frontal lobe is necessary for speaking and the right frontal lobe holds our sense of humour. You can appreciate that frontal lobe damage can often seem to change a person.

Deep within the hemispheres lie the **basal ganglia**, which are involved in performing movements, and the **limbic system**, which generates our emotions. All these different parts of the brain are connected by long fibres called **axons**, but which are often simply referred to as 'white matter'. This enables really effective communication so that parts of the brain can work together in harmony.

Damage to different parts of the brain results in different outcomes. For example, a stroke in the occipital lobe would result in someone having significant visual problems, while stroke damage to the cerebellum will affect balance; damage to the areas that process memories would cause forgetfulness.

My bleed was predominantly in the white matter, the connections, alongside the basal ganglia in the right hemisphere. When Helen was first told of the damage to my brain she was relieved that there seemed to be little harm to the actual lobes of my cerebrum, but she had not appreciated that the connections that link these different parts of the brain are also crucial to brain functioning. The damage that I suffered meant that messages were no longer reliably transmitted to and from different parts of my brain on the right side and this caused problems because it meant that key parts of my brain, even though they were reasonably intact, were no longer activated or coordinated.

The brain can be likened to an orchestra where efficient communication is absolutely necessary for the coordination of different parts of the ensemble. If the coordination is poor in an orchestra the music sounds terrible; if the coordination within the brain is poor, then all sorts of functions can be disrupted. My right brain could no longer reliably transmit messages and therefore the complicated (but usually seamless) interacting of the different parts of my brain was messed up and the result of this was that I initially struggled with a whole range of things: my vision, my speech, my movement, my ability to concentrate, to 'think straight' and to problem solve and plan. Some of my abilities to reason and to curb impulses (abilities that lay in my undamaged frontal lobes) just weren't available to me after the stroke and I am told that I was quite unlike my usual reserved, professorial self for a while. It is encouraging that over time these connections have steadily (if slowly) recovered, my concentration and thinking processes in general have much improved and my family is relieved to have the 'old Udo' back again.

By now I think I've made the point that the outcome of a stroke will be determined by the area of the brain that is damaged. My stroke was on the right side, so I kept my language skills, but my spatial abilities are poor even two years later and it will probably always be a challenge for me to imagine things in 3D or to find my way around inside an unfamiliar building.

Interestingly my 'left-brain' abilities seemed even better than before, and much to my wife's irritation I pedantically correct her grammar and finish her sentences. I began doing this within a day or two of my stroke and I haven't really let up on her since.

By far the most obvious sign of my stroke being in the right side of my brain was my left-sided paralysis. My left leg and arm were useless immediately after my stroke. This is known as **hemi-paresis** or **hemiplegia** when there is no movement at all. In the first days after my stroke, I slept most of the time, and I have only snippets of memories from this period. My wife, who visited me daily, told me that on admission I was able to debate the nature of the injury to my brain with my colleagues, so I was lucid and verbal, yet my left arm and leg were completely immobile. When I was able to talk about my physical experience I described myself as no longer having a sense of being a whole person. I was not simply weakened in my left side – it was as if my left side was no longer part of me.

Something else happened as a result of my brain being damaged on the right side: I neglected the entire left side of my surroundings. I stopped taking notice of it; it was as if it didn't exist. This is common after strokes in the right side of the brain and is called **hemi-neglect**. And it went beyond my own body – if I had two visitors I would only attend to the one on my right. I only noted my other visitor (on my left) if they actively drew my attention – I recall my sister, who had travelled from Germany, waving and shouting, 'I've come all this way – look at me!'

Sometimes I would be aware of what happened, or was happening, to my left but only when someone brought it to my notice.

One afternoon Helen came into my hospital room saying: 'Didn't you hear me knocking on your door?'

'Yes,' I replied, because when she pointed it out, I realised that I had heard her knocking but it had been just a background noise that didn't really seem to matter. It was like having the experience of walking with a bird-watching friend who every now and then says: 'There's a blackbird singing.' You realise that you had been hearing birdsong but not fully noticing it, and in my case not finding it particularly important. The aspect of hemi-neglect that amused my children was evident at mealtimes when I would clear the food only on the right side of the plate, leaving a perfect half-circle of uneaten dinner on the left, quite careless of the fact that I had half a meal waiting to be consumed. They took it upon themselves to wait, watch, chuckle at my expense and then twist my plate around so that I could 'see' the rest of my meal and finish eating.

Had my bleed been on the left side of my brain then my hemi-neglect might have been for the right side of my environment. However, the parts of the brain that help us attend to things are predominantly in the right side of the brain so damage to the right hemisphere is more likely to cause hemi-neglect. If someone has damage to the left side of the brain they might suffer from right hemi-neglect, but it is much less common and when it does occur it is often more easily overcome, so that is good news for some.

To make things even more difficult in my case, the right-sided bleed caused **left-sided hemianopia**. This means that I was blind in my left fields of vision in each eye. What I saw was a great black hole to my left, jagged round the edge, deep and dark. I could only see the left side of faces or the endings of words or just that one side of my plate. This happens because the messages from the eye to the brain are disrupted by the stroke. A hemianopia from a left-brain stroke would have given me blindness in my right visual field. Fortunately, and this is typical, the hemianopia gradually disappeared. After three weeks I only had a quarter of my vision missing (this is called **quadrantanopia**) and then after about six weeks my vision cleared, and I had no blindness at all. In addition, the hemi-neglect improved somewhat with rehabilitation – although it is still there and when I'm tired it gets worse; in fact, it is one of the tell-tale signs that I need to rest.

When I worked as a medical consultant I often encountered people who had suffered damage to their left brain and who had lost their ability to use language. This is different from loss of speech as speech loss (or **dysarthria**) is usually related to loss of the muscle control necessary to form sounds and this can occur with right- or left-hemisphere damage. We use one hundred muscles when we speak – muscles that help us articulate our words but also muscles that force air through our voice box. I had severe muscle weakness on my left side following my stroke so no wonder that my speech became slurred and quiet and I had difficulty swallowing. I'm lucky in that I now have no difficulties speaking or swallowing, although my voice is much quieter than it used to be, and I have had to accept that I simply no longer have the muscle power to talk loudly.

Loss of language is a more complicated phenomenon and is always related to damage to the left side of the brain. Some people lose the ability to understand language (spoken and written), others lose the ability to express themselves in words and sadly some people lose both aspects of language. I can only imagine the trauma of suffering a stroke and then having the additional shock of not being able to understand anything that is being said, not being able to take any comfort or instruction, and this sometimes being compounded by a total inability to express oneself.

In her TED Talk, 'My Stroke of Insight', Dr Jill Bolte Taylor describes the morning that she suffered a left-sided stroke. As a neuroscientist she recognised what was happening. At first, she seemed calm and she was simply curious about her experience, but then she decided to phone a colleague for help. This was not easy as she could no longer remember her office phone number and when she tried to look it up, she found that she couldn't recognise letters and numbers – they were just pixels to her now. Miraculously she managed to make the call, and, in her mind, she was describing her predicament clearly but what her colleague heard was gobbledegook and what she heard when he replied was gobbledegook. She had lost the ability to read, to speak and to hear language but, and this is an important but, just a few years later she was giving a very articulate TED Talk.

I have seen the frustration and distress that loss of language can cause both the patient and their loved ones, but I have also seen people relearn language and speech and even those who could not speak learnt other ways to reconnect with people around them, by gestures and facial expressions. So again, it is reasonable to hold on to hope and it is important to make full use of available speech and language therapy services so that any potential to communicate can be fulfilled.

What happens immediately after the stroke?

A newly damaged brain is vulnerable and the first days and even weeks after a stroke are crucial periods where close watch is kept because of the risk of further strokes or epileptic fits. As time passes the risk of stroke or fits will decrease and it is in these early days that the most rapid recovery is made as swellings in the brain subside. The swellings usually come from the blood that gathers after a brain bleed (a **haematoma**) and from the swelling that typically surrounds damaged tissues (an **oedema**).

As you now know, I had a bleeding in my brain – a haematoma – and as this worsened it pressed on my brain tissue, crushing the surrounding brain cells. Sometimes the neurosurgeons decide that it is necessary to operate in order to relieve the pressure of the bleed, sometimes they decide against it as they did in my case. However, once the bleeding has stopped, the blood will slowly be reabsorbed by the body's normal cleaning-up mechanisms. So, if you were able to look at my brain scans over the months following my stroke you would see the haematoma getting smaller and as it did you would notice my condition improving.

Following any damage to tissue there is usually a swelling, and the brain is no exception. As the oedema develops around the injured part of the brain it increases the pressure within the skull and this can cause not just swelling but pain and even further damage, much as a brain bleed can. Perhaps mercifully I have little recollection of the first few days following my stroke, but my wife remembers vividly the head pain that I experienced in the first forty-eight hours, pain that was attributed to oedema in addition to the bleed. Even though I was given very powerful painkillers I still rated my headaches as 9/10 for severity. Once again, neurosurgeons kept a close eye on me and ultimately decided not to operate to relieve the pressure. Just as with the haematoma, after the swelling has stopped the body will usually reabsorb the excess fluid, the swelling and discomfort will ease, and a patient will show signs of recovery.

What recovery can we expect?

This is possibly the most common question but a hard one to answer. When a doctor isn't able to give you a precise answer she or he is not being awkward; the fact is that no two stroke survivors will make quite the same recovery because no two brains are the same, no two strokes are the same and the surroundings in which recovery takes place vary enormously. However, we can say with confidence that proper rehabilitation will help a person reach their recovery potential and we can say with confidence that in a month's time we'll see some recovery and in six months' time we will see even more recovery – we just can't say how much.

I had a long time in a hospital bed contemplating 'What is a stroke?' but even on the very first day I realised that although I'd been a stroke specialist for over twenty years there was so much that I hadn't known. The things that I had read and observed as a doctor were only part of appreciating what it is like to suffer brain damage and to try to rebuild a meaningful life. I really feel that I am now more of a specialist than I ever was. So, the rest of this book is dedicated to sharing my enriched learning, along with our family's experiences, in the hope that it will help you better cope and emerge from this potentially life-changing event.

2

The Early Days: Shock and Fear

The day of the stroke will probably be etched in the memories of anyone who experiences one either as the victim or as someone who cares for the victim. For us the trauma began the night before. Udo, an otherwise healthy sixty-two-year-old with low blood pressure, ran as hard as he'd ever run to catch the last train home from Wolverhampton. As he settled in his train seat, he was aware that something had happened, he'd experienced severe head pain and he felt weakened on the left side. It crossed his mind that he'd had a stroke. Nonetheless, he felt calm and the pain and weakness faded so he continued his journey home. He reached Oxford, hailed a taxi, climbed the steps into the house and joined Helen for a brief conversation before she went to bed and he sat at the PC to unwind.

Sometime in the early hours of the morning the bleed deep in his brain that must have begun in Wolverhampton enlarged enough for him to pass out and it now invaded a large area of his right hemisphere, leaving him paralysed and blind on his left side. Helen found him on the floor of the study, lying beside a broken chair, at 7 a.m. on Sunday 9 October 2016.

By then he was conscious and had been trying for some hours to cry out and get up, but his voice and his body were weak. From the moment that he regained consciousness the calm of the previous night had disappeared and was replaced by terror. He couldn't move his left side, nor could he use his right side to push himself up from the floor. Why couldn't he push himself up? He was shocked and bewildered by his physical helplessness. Why was his right side not working properly either? Only later did he appreciate that his left side was not just weakened and without sensation, it no longer felt a part of him: he was now a man with only a right side and he had lost the sense of where the mid-line of his body should be. This meant that he could no longer judge how to push himself into a sitting position and he could no longer coordinate the necessary movements even though his right side still functioned. All he could do was panic and wait to be found.

He had quickly diagnosed his own stroke, so he gave his wife precise instructions to call the ambulance. Also filled with panic, she raced through the house, shouting to our sixteen-year-old daughter: 'Dad's had a stroke – ambulance on the way – quick, get up – I need help!' On reflection this was not the way to spread the news, traumatising a teen who should have heard it in a measured and thoughtful way. But we all make mistakes under stress and this wouldn't be the last – and as you'll see our family survived, each of us falling short of perfection over and over again. Families are like that.

Despite the shock of what we had just suffered, we also knew that we were lucky. Udo had his stroke in Oxford where the medical care is nearby; had this happened a few months earlier he might have been abroad, far from the nearest hospital and he might not have lived. We were also lucky that he had a right-hemisphere bleed, so he was able to speak and communicate, albeit in a quiet and slurred fashion. We were lucky that he'd been found before 8 a.m. when the Oxford City roads closed in preparation for the annual half-marathon. We were very lucky that he was cared for by colleagues at the John Radcliffe Hospital, Oxford, where he often worked. 'But this is Udo!' stressed a consultant in A&E, and we knew we were in good hands. At that time, it helped to hang on to all the reasons for feeling fortunate because there was bad news, too.

'It's a big bleed.'

'How big?'

'The size of a clenched fist . . .'

The chance of surviving such a large intracerebral bleed was less than 50 per cent. Udo knew this better than most and he decided to keep that information to himself.

For many, recollections of such a day will be hazy and fragmented. That's the nature of traumatic memories. For us, time became distorted, certain events stood out, other things were forgotten. There is no point in anguishing over remembering it right, we often can't. But what we are left with is a general 'gist' for that day with some vivid recall. We both recalled the repeated medical phrase, 'Sluggish response', which scared Helen. But we also remembered the reassurance that, 'We won't operate on Udo unless it's absolutely necessary – and we are neurosurgeons, Helen, we like to operate', which gave us reassurance and hope as well as a weak smile. Anyone who has been through this will have good and bad fragments of memory. Hold on to the good, so that the recollection of that day is not just steeped in terror.

Within the first hour Udo discussed his precise diagnosis with his former colleagues. The results shown on the scans ('. . . a large intracerebral bleed in the area of the right basal ganglia') fitted with his physical experience of severe left-sided weakness – so severe that he could not move, and the left side of his face had become twisted. This made medical sense to Udo and he drew some comfort from his medical world still being in order.

From A&E, we moved up to the Neurology Intensive Care Unit (NICU). This was a familiar area for us. It had been a sometime place of work for Udo, but it had also been the unit that had cared for a dear friend who had suffered a brain bleed three years earlier. Our friend survived and made good progress. Indeed, he was back at work as a solicitor within six months: we hung on to that hope, that Udo might recover and resume his work as a doctor. Hang on to hope even if expectations and plans need to be revised later.

Day one was a day of Udo sleeping, intensive checking, a day of tubes and procedures. For Helen it was a day of feeling detached from reality. For our children it was a day of neglect, just receiving the odd text that managed to make its way out of the hospital. Caught up in the intensity of the crisis Helen kept forgetting the fears and needs of the fourteen- and sixteen-year-old at home.

To be fair, holding this bigger picture of the family was difficult with Udo passing in and out of consciousness and fearful questions dominating our thinking: *Will he survive? If he does, will he be himself? If he is, will he walk?*

Sitting by a hospital bed Helen thought about herself and Udo, sometimes losing sight of the family as a whole – just when the kids needed to be held and supported. Later this realisation provided excellent fodder for self-criticism, but reproach is an additional burden on a person who is struggling to cope, and the reality is that we are human and we all make mistakes. We have good intentions, we do the best we can, and we sometimes fall short of the mark – it is regrettable but understandable. We've since apologised and explained as best we could to the kids and discovered that they were accepting and compassionate – an example to their parents, in fact.

There are memories of professionals that stand out because they saw the bigger picture – seeing beyond the patient. On that first day a very kind NICU consultant brought a real coffee and a pecan slice to a bewildered wife sitting by the bedside of a man who had once again drifted into some other realm. It was a kindness that gave much needed strength that went beyond the caffeine-kick. Later an NICU nurse sensed Helen's need for respite and appreciated that the teens at home might need their mum. She reassured Helen that Udo was stable, that there was little to be done now and it was okay to take some time out. Without her clear reassurances it would have been hard to leave Udo's side, but she saw that it was the best thing for our family.

By now the cocktail of intravenous medications had begun: mainly steroids to reduce the swelling in the brain, anti-hypertensives to lower blood pressure, morphine for the headaches and anticonvulsants to prevent epileptic fits. The effect of this was to make Udo quite woozy and playful and as he and Helen sat together in the evening just before she left he whispered: 'You have to admit that I bring you to the most romantic places.'

On day two he was not so playful. As his brain swelled following its trauma, the headaches worsened, his blood pressure spiked, and he was under close observation and spent most of the time sleeping. Helen was now joined by our daughter, a courageous young woman. We know how courageous she was because we had seen an essay that she had written after visiting our friend three years earlier. As part of her schoolwork she had been asked to share her most frightening memory – it was her visit to the NICU. She wrote about the haunting 'Beep. Beep. Hiss . . .' of the hospital equipment and her initial impression of the unit:

> . . . I followed her into the ICU, the limbo of the living world; the most depressing place I have ever encountered. A crypt of occupied hospital beds, inhabited by seemingly lifeless bodies, surrounded by friends and family members who stare blankly at the person they used to love or hate . . .

Back then we had assumed that, at thirteen, our daughter would be able to tolerate the hospital environment – after all, she had been into work with her father on several occasions. But on the day of that visit she had taken her father's arm as she walked into the unit and had told him that she was scared, very scared. She had only kept going so that she could support her friend. Her brother was fourteen when Udo had the stroke and we did not press him to visit now we understood how traumatic the NICU can be, especially when the patient is your own father.

That second day was harder: more real. Witnessing our children's distress, seeing Udo in such pain, fearing that he would need surgery, contacting people to let them know, sitting amongst the 'Beep. Beep. Hiss . . .' of our daughter's nightmare. It all began to bring home the significance of the stroke. Udo ate nothing and slept 90 per cent of the time and we were told, 'This is what he needs – it's normal.' These reassurances reminded us that so many of the odd behaviours and reactions are 'normal' in these 'abnormal' circumstances and we needed to know that.

In his brief waking moments Udo was back with us fiercely debating his diagnosis. With good reasoning, he thought that he might have suffered an ischaemic stroke prior to the bleed and he would maintain this point then suddenly fall into a deep sleep, sometimes halfway through a sentence. This was particularly unnerving for his daughter who'd never seen Dad like this and Helen wished that she had prepared her better – but there was so little time for planning.

By day three we were hearing the term 'stable' even though the headaches were more severe, and temperature and blood pressure were raised. Morphine seemed to offer little relief. An unwelcome nasal tube joined others invading Udo's body. He was strong enough to argue against this medical decision but too weak to fight it.

When Udo was conscious he continued to complain of worsening headaches. Helen assumed the worst, namely that the bleeding deep in his brain was continuing, and she feared for his life. However, the surgeons kept a close eye on him and they maintained that surgery wasn't necessary. It was very likely not bleeding causing the headache but the swelling of the brain that follows a stroke. Just as we get a swelling around an injured limb, we get swelling round an injured brain. This continued for days but it eventually subsided, and the headaches did improve.

On day four Udo moved to the dedicated Stroke Unit within the same hospital. This was hopeful because it showed that he was stable enough to leave NICU, although he still struggled with the headaches and his voice was little more than a whisper. The NICU had been the realm of regular beeps and hisses; the Stroke Unit was the realm of jostling, hoisting and unpredictable noise. The patients were four to a room and more vociferous than the occupants of the NICU, but Udo could now tolerate this and was thus making progress.

Udo's first consultant on the Stroke Unit was someone who knew him professionally, and she called him 'Professor' from the outset, a thoughtful gesture that gave him dignity and elevated him from disabled patient to the person he was. As we were to come to appreciate more and more, it is so important not to lose sight of the person and the therapeutic power of dignity.

Not everyone dignified Udo, though. Around this time, he explained to his daughter: 'My stroke affects my voice and makes me sound like an old man.'

'No, Dad, being an old man makes you sound like an old man.'

No dignity, but very welcome playfulness.

In a waking moment he told Helen that he was a 'Level One Patient', which meant that he knew that he was severely disabled by his stroke and would need intensive rehabilitation. He was wholly immobile, needing to be hoisted regularly, and he was not even able to swallow. He was fed via a tube that went through his nose straight into his stomach.

At this time, he was literally half blind with hemianopia. His left field of vision was missing so a word such as 'soft' appeared as '-ft' and a sentence such as: 'The rain in Spain' read as '-he -ain -n -ain'. We realised that he had this condition when he looked up and said: 'Darling, you have only one eye.' He had assumed that he knew what this must be like for the patient – after all, he'd read the books – but he was not prepared for the shock of his own experience. When he looked down at his hands on his lap, there was not simply a one-sided clouding of his visual field as he'd expected but a deep black hole with jagged red edges that swallowed up his left hand or his phone when he put it into his left pocket. Worst was looking at people because half of their face would disappear into a jagged black hole, making them look like something from a horror film. It was especially distressing to see loved ones like this and made it harder for him to draw much-needed comfort from their visits. For the first time in his career he properly appreciated the distress of hemianopia.

At this time, he still had no active movement or sensation to touch or awareness in his left leg or arm. He knew this as hemiparesis and he was profoundly shocked by it. He experienced more than simply numbness and paralysis; it was as if his left side no longer belonged to his body. He would look at his left arm and instead of owning it, he was reminded of his time in the medical school mortuary because it was a detached and lifeless limb to him. When he woke in the night his right hand would feel his cold left arm and it seemed like a dead body part lying across him. This was so real in the lonely early hours of the morning that Udo would even worry about the limb decomposing, which added to the horror of it all.

The distress of perceiving one's own arm as a dead limb or a world of black holes can make a person doubt their sanity and Udo now wondered if his own patients had not described such experiences to him for fear of seeming crazy. He was also beginning to realise that he'd rarely encouraged them to talk about their experiences in such detail. Typically, he listened long enough to diagnose the problem and then would move into what he called his 'doctor mode', aiming to give relief as quickly as possible by explaining the condition and describing the prognosis and the treatment. This was done with the best intention but if he had his time over again he would have been more curious about each individual's experiences and he would have been better prepared to understand the fears of some of his patients.

He also had another condition, hemi-neglect, whereby he became unaware of his left side. It wasn't that he couldn't 'see' to his left, his left side no longer had any relevance for him. Nothing to his left side had real substance; it was often absent from his consciousness and events to his left didn't matter to Udo. Typical of patients with hemi-neglect, the condition didn't trouble him: after all, the left side was irrelevant so why should it worry him? It tended to bother others more; it certainly bothered his wife and children. At visiting time, we would knock on his door (which was to his left) only to be ignored and when we did enter his room he would only address the person on his right; the others would have to work hard to be noticed. We didn't realise this at first and so when we visited at least one of us would feel ignored and unimportant. Also because of the hemi-neglect, Udo would only look to his right to locate an object. He would no longer consider scanning his left side, so others had to find his 'missing' books or his phone, which was sometimes a cause for family irritation. While he still had the hemianopia, one friend got used to prompting him with the phrase: 'Look in the black hole, Udo' – a reminder to search the left side of his world – and so often he'd then find his phone or some other object.

And there was yet another odd aspect to his hemi-neglect: when given instructions or messages from his left side he tended not to take them in. Thus, a person would leave the room (from Udo's left) bidding him farewell and a few minutes later Udo still assumed that they were present. This happened despite attempts to make exits memorable with exaggerated arm-waving and repeated goodbyes. Over the following months, Helen lost count of the number of times her phone would ring on the way home and it would be Udo asking her to fetch him something because he had not registered her leaving and he assumed that she was still in the hospital. While Helen and the kids were upset each time this happened, Udo considered it the least of his problems and sometimes even felt annoyed when it was raised as a concern.

After the initial shock of the stroke, followed by the relief that a loved one has survived, a new fear sometimes emerges – the fear that the loved one has changed and is lost. Conditions such as hemi-neglect, hemianopia and hemiparesis can result in such odd responses that it might seem as though the patient is no longer themselves and this can be heartbreaking and terrifying for the family, particularly the younger members. This was the case for us. Now that Udo was on the Stroke Unit he could more easily receive visitors, so we went as a whole family and our son saw his dad for the first time since the stroke.

The Stroke Unit was at the end of a long, cold corridor lined with abandoned medical equipment that could look quite sinister, not a comfortable walk for the nervous, and young visitors can be very nervous. Simply entering a ward is often unsettling for the hospital naïve and looking back we wished we'd better prepared our kids by talking things through more and perhaps showing them a photo or two of their father in the hospital bed. In our defence, those first few days were a blur of trying to cope and we weren't the best project managers. A wise friend – more 'with it' than us at the time – suggested we meet her outside the ward before going in to see Dad. This meant that there was another friendly person for support and to ease things, which it did.

The ward, like so many in the NHS, was a beehive of activity and there was a sense of efficiency – which was comforting to Helen – but there was little sense of calming and there was little that was uplifting, which was what our kids needed. We were bustled into the busy four-bedded room and our son was immediately faced by his father slumped in a bed, weak and pale with a distorted face. The teen was silent, but his distress was palpable. It didn't get easier for him and silent weeks and weeks followed. Only later did we learn that he had been so shocked by Udo's appearance that he believed that his dad must be dying, but he kept his fears to himself – for the next two years.

Udo now received many visitors, even though most of the time they would be observing a sleeping friend. Nonetheless, in his short periods of waking his spirits lifted when visitors were present, and he chatted coherently, grateful for the care that he was receiving and already discussing his plans to write about his experiences so that he might help fellow rehabilitationists. In the first week these brief episodes of communication gave us hope for the future: Udo was still with us, a thoughtful person and a dedicated doctor. We dared to hope that we'd get through this crisis and get back to normal.

We visited as often as possible and Helen began dousing herself in Chanel No. 5 and wearing stripy sweaters to help him quickly recognise her in his half-blind and distractible state because he was so cheered when he realised that his wife had arrived. Indeed, he so was grateful for the kind attention of any friends and staff that he became overly effusive in his thanks and over a period of days his gratitude began to dominate his conversation to the extent that staff encouraged him to limit his thankyous. This was the beginning of a disturbing phase of *excessive* gratitude that was untypical of Udo and the first sign of changes in him. These were changes that his son quickly picked up and they unnerved the boy even more. Perhaps it was a blessing that there was also much else going on during visits: the parallel conversations in the shared room, the frequent brief reviews by professionals and the arrival of hospital meals all served as welcome distractions for our teens.

In A&E, a consultant had told Helen that Udo would need 'heavy-duty rehab' so it was good to see that among the early visitors were therapists: speech therapists to help with swallowing of very soft foods, physiotherapists to aid sitting and occupational therapists checking out attention span and hemi-neglect. Rehabilitation had begun, and it felt as though we were now properly on the road to recovery. Our friend, a neuropsychologist, suggested that there should now be a sign over Udo's bed saying: 'Do not administer psychological tests: this patient knows the answers.'

However, the headaches were no better and there was no noticeable physical progress. We kept being told that he was 'stable'. Once this had been reassuring but now it was worrying – we wanted to hear 'progress'. Having said this, it was good that we weren't given false hope and we learnt to appreciate that. The challenge from now on was to keep that balance of hope but not false hope.

Days passed in the hospital. There was no observable improvement and Helen became sadder. She thought that Udo was too because of his tearfulness but he explained that this was simply 'emotional lability', typical following a brain injury. This means that a person is very easily moved to tears and it is sometimes called 'pathological crying' or, rather insensitively, 'emotional incontinence'. Udo easily became tearful in conversations about moving issues or when watching poignant scenes in films and quite often laughter would morph into tears. He was familiar with this phenomenon as it is common in stroke patients but that didn't make it any easier to tolerate, especially by a man who had formerly been the emotionally calm and stoical consultant to the people who were now caring for him.

At this time Udo, so grateful for his survival and the love and support he received, spoke repeatedly of his wonderful wife and the centrality of his family, which of course triggered tears. These were sentiments that we knew he held but we weren't used to such effusive expression and certainly not in front of strangers. So, despite the satisfaction of hearing him speak so lovingly, we were somewhat discomfited by these uncharacteristic public pronouncements. As time went on we witnessed more uncharacteristic behaviours. For example, Udo very rarely swore and on the first day of the stroke as he reflected on his experience of semi-paralysis, hemi-neglect and hemianopia he uttered a phrase that he was to repeat over the next few weeks: 'For over twenty years I've been advising people on stroke and I knew bugger all!' This became such a frequent – but also very pertinent – utterance that at one point we considered it as the subtitle for this book.

There were other behaviours that were exaggerated and pressing. One evening Helen arrived and Udo had mentally composed a lengthy letter to *Empire* magazine because he was so outraged that it had not given the film *The Magnificent Seven* a better rating. With an urgency rarely before seen, he insisted that the letter be typed and retyped and e-mailed and when it wasn't possible that night he carried on the urgent demand the next day, and the next. He somehow rang home in the early hours to summon Helen to come to the hospital to perfect the e-mail. He wouldn't let it go; it was as if he couldn't let it drop. And of course, he couldn't, his frontal lobes were not working properly and without their help we become inflexible in our thinking and fixed on ideas.

Such unusual behaviours are usual when the brain is swollen and especially when brain damage is in the area of Udo's stroke, but it can be difficult for loved ones to adjust to and it is sometimes embarrassing for the patient to look back on. We were fortunate that our friends and Udo's carers did not particularly draw attention to these changes and we were lucky that he never did anything that he later felt uneasy about, but Udo had seen many people during his career who had behaved in ways that were shocking and it is as well to be prepared and not be too judgemental towards the patient. We saw staff in the Stroke Unit doing this beautifully – achieving a balance of being firm but kind and not drawing attention to conduct that might otherwise pave a pathway to shame.

In these early days the cards and letters began to arrive – friends, colleagues, patients, all sending best wishes but also reminding Udo of his valuable role as a doctor. Although it would become a source of anguish – would Udo ever be able to return to medical work? – at this time of severe disability it was heartening to be reminded of the value of the person in the hospital bed. Of course, all these expressions of admiration triggered emotional lability and with every card came another cascade of tears. But not just from Udo: Helen often matched him tear-for-tear because the messages were so very touching.

The early days in particular are a time of upheaval and it is bewildering for spouse and children so the few discussions we had with medical staff were very welcome. It's easy to become fazed or catastrophic and just a few words from staff can be orientating. It's often difficult to retain these words of wisdom and solace so you might want to take notes or even record conversations on your phone – as long as you have agreement from the professional, of course.

Sadly, in busy NHS units, despite best efforts, there is often too little time for the family members who also need support. Our kids struggled – both wanted to be with their father, but not under these conditions. Both could 'see' their father, but he wasn't their dad right now. His face was twisted; his speech slow, sometimes inaudible; and he held strange, sentimental conversations that triggered tears. This was especially difficult for two teens who had only recently graduated from being very bonded to Mum and had begun forging a close relationship with their father. They missed him, and this would last for weeks that turned into months.

We were offered family support. If you have the same opportunity, we would encourage you to consider this early on even though we didn't. We decided not to because the children felt too close to some of the staff in the unit and Helen felt awkward about accepting such personal support from people who were not quite friends, but who were closer to us than the average professional. She began to appreciate the challenge that lay ahead for Udo, who had no choice but to accept his friends and colleagues as his professional helpers. We were again lucky in that one of our closest friends was an expert in supporting young persons with a parent with brain injury. She would find time to join Helen and the children for informal suppers where she skilfully helped the teens come to terms with the new situation by uncovering some of their fears and then allaying them with assurances that there would be progress, we just couldn't say how much at this stage.

She also gave Helen a valuable piece of advice, which was not to burden the kids with responsibility for their dad. It is easy to look to older children in particular and ask them to take on caretaking roles, but this might be a time when they've not got the emotional resources to do so. Also, we risk undermining the sense of security that comes from knowing that Mum and Dad are there for them in this time of crisis. So, as parents, we made it clear in those early days that we didn't expect the children to take on a carer's role at all, but Helen was also clear that if either of them wanted to help her out and support her in practical ways she'd be most grateful. They both stepped up to the mark – leaving Mum to be responsible for Dad but helping out with domestic chores and proffering plenty of hugs.

By day ten we heard the phrase 'stable' every day, but we were still not hearing 'progress'. And it is true that there was little change. Sleep still predominated, the paralysis and visual impairment seemed no better but the next move was about to happen.

On 20 October, Udo was transferred to the Oxford Centre of Enablement, a specialist neuro-rehabilitation unit with an excellent reputation and formerly the workplace of one Professor Udo Kischka.

3

Beginning Rehabilitation: 'Who Are You and What Have You Done with My Dad?'

A great deal of thought had gone into Udo's move to the O.C.E. We had considered the pros and cons of his being in an excellent local unit, but one run by colleagues. The staff had also considered the pros and cons – wanting to give Udo the best treatment but being aware of the potential awkwardness of this. On balance we, Udo and Helen, decided that the O.C.E. was the best choice and the staff stepped up to the mark brilliantly.

From the outset the hospital atmosphere changed. Previous professional carers had on the whole been friendly and capable but at the O.C.E. there was palpable warmth from Udo's colleagues. There were also important physical changes as he now had a single room with en-suite bathroom – so much more dignified than only having flimsy curtains for privacy. To improve matters further, he left behind the smooth, pink yoghurts of the previous unit and could now eat lumpy, 'manly' food as he called it. We felt a surge of optimism even though Udo remained 'stable' and we saw no progress beyond the shift from pink to 'manly' food. His optimism came from a firm belief: 'The brain is remarkable, and neuro-rehabilitation can achieve great things.'

Looking back, Udo was perhaps over-optimistic about his progress in these early days, but this outlook gave him hope and with that came the motivation to work at his recovery. Some of the staff had told us that 'motivation is nine-tenths of rehabilitation', so at least we had that going for us.

Frequently we were told to 'expect a marathon not a sprint', indicating the slow pattern of progress. This is a fair statement, but no one can tell you when and if you'll reach the finishing line and our experience was that the finishing line kept moving further away as the months in the O.C.E. stretched on. So, the reassurance of the marathon metaphor weakened for us. Another phrase we heard was: 'Recovery will be a roller-coaster', and this is true insofar as the ups and downs are often extreme. For our tenth wedding anniversary we had revisited Disneyland where we'd married a decade earlier. One particular ride there, California Screaming, turned out to be a favourite for father and daughter. This was a magnificent roller-coaster that looped back as well as driving forwards. For us this is what Udo's roller-coaster progress was like: he didn't just go up and down in his journey, but he regularly slipped back. An infection, of which there were several, would set him back for a week or two or more; similarly, fatigue or low blood pressure would take its toll. So extreme was one of the setbacks caused by infection that his brain was re-scanned to check that he had not suffered another bleed.

The past days (and the days to come) had given us stress without respite and our emotional state was fragile. This meant that the roller-coaster was an internal experience, too. Emotions soared and swooped. At the end of a day we could be buoyed up by hope because there had been a twitch of a muscle or a glimmer of the old Udo or we could be crushed by despair because the old Udo had disappeared again, or we discovered that the twitch was an involuntary spasm. One of the most impressive involuntary spasms was the bending and raising of his left arm during a yawn. Udo looked like Napoleon in pyjamas.

We experienced many bouts of regression over the months – and still do. As you read through our account of the first two years following Udo's stroke you will see that the ups and downs and setbacks have become part of our lives because a damaged brain remains a vulnerable brain. This takes its toll on the family, so you will also see that we get burnt out from time to time and we

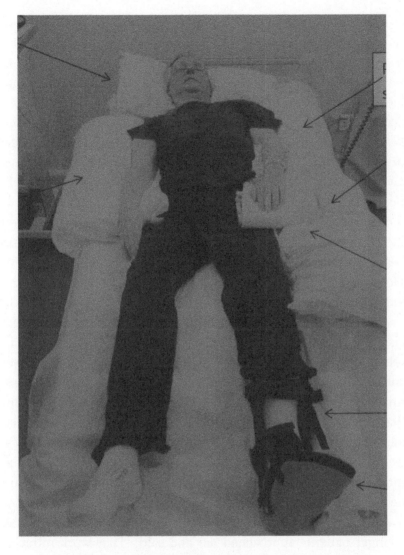

At the O.C.E. in the early days. Unable to support himself,
Udo relies on pillows and splints

sometimes feel profoundly helpless, particularly Udo. We consciously had to remind ourselves that we could forge something better – and it does get better, but in these early days and in the weeks and sometimes months to come you might need to brace yourself for a very rough ride.

A damaged brain has fewer reserves than a whole brain, so it will quickly show signs of stress and strain. It is demoralising and frightening when this happens but standing back and trying to review our overall progress helped whenever things seemed too bleak. Around the time of the move to the O.C.E. Helen began keeping a daily log and the entries over the days and weeks helped keep the longer-term picture in mind and allowed us to review progress. It was also a cathartic outpouring alone in the evenings and it was a connection to Udo as it was written to him. The loneliness within the family of the stroke victim can be intense: gone is the companion and help-mate, the person who would have been the support in this crisis. Even though we did have places and people to turn to we often had the feeling of nowhere to go. For Helen, a written nocturnal dialogue with Udo eased this, while the kids drifted into a make-believe world delivered by the internet.

At the end of the first day at the O.C.E. our feelings were mixed: elated that Udo was still alive and now stable enough to be in rehab and hopeful that this would restore him back to us, yet sobered at the sight of him drifting in and out of awareness, unable to sit and constantly slithering down the pillow mountain that supported him, his unfamiliar twisted face looking bemused and helpless – which indeed he was. Bemusement was now a frequent state of mind for Udo as the world went by a bit too quickly and he didn't always catch the drift of conversations and he was still so very, very tired.

As Helen left the unit that night the mother of one of the younger patients approached her and said: 'They work miracles here. This is the miracle hospital.' This is what we needed to hear, we felt that we needed a miracle. In his time as a consultant at the O.C.E. Udo had seen many miracles achieved in this unit and he had a strong belief that this place would deliver.

In these early days Udo had brief periods of being aware, very aware, but sadly he was not 'with it' for most of the time. Things frequently went over his head – and no wonder as his brain was swollen and his sleep broken. Our sense of having lost the person that we knew as Udo grew now that he spent more time awake. This is what prompted our daughter to ask: 'Who are you and what have you done with my dad?' This was meant affectionately, to tease a smile from him, but there was a sobering subtext. His kindly lopsided face almost constantly turned to the right, his 'good' side, was that of an almost stranger. And now that he spoke more, the change in him was amplified by a twisted mouth and slurred speech. There were also physical changes for the kids to adjust to: his useless left hand began to balloon with fluid retention and in its tight compression glove it looked like a haggis with fingers. At the same time his left ankle became swollen and disfigured. He could not support himself, so he was strapped into a specialist wheel-chair with a headrest and high sides. He needed to wear hand and ankle splints and he still sported invasive tubes. Although we knew that all these aids were absolutely necessary, Udo felt diminished by them and they made him look even less like himself.

Finally, the environment took away his role as a doctor – he was a patient now and well and truly not his former self. But painful as it was to witness it was crucial that we accepted things had changed so that he could do what is so very difficult for a doctor: he could fully become a patient, tolerating the discomforts and sometimes indignities that go with it.

Having said that, there was so much that staff did to minimise the indignities. Half paralysed and wholly weak, Udo was unable to do the simplest things and needed to be hoisted from bed to wheelchair. He felt undignified and embarrassed dangling in mid-air, his already shrinking body diminishing further as he was swallowed by the hoist sheet. Sensing this, a particularly thought-ful nurse smiled and said: 'Welcome to NHS Airlines, your flight attendants will be . . .' and the tension was defused. This was one of many instances of expert staff helping Udo smile in the face of adversity whilst retaining dignity and camaraderie. Throughout his career he had avoided using humour with patients. He had been concerned that they might feel he was trivialising their predicament, but he discovered that humour can be uplifting and motivating if it's used sensitively and within a respectful relationship.

We soon discovered that the profound helplessness, new to Udo, shifted his fear threshold dramatically. He felt so helpless that the most benign things triggered panic. His greatest fear was falling and having another brain bleed, but other seemingly innocuous things were a source of great worry too. A misplaced cushion: 'What if I get pain?'; the new wooden handrail: 'What if I get a splinter?'; going for a short jaunt in the fresh air: 'What if I get cold?', 'What if you roll the wheelchair over?', 'What if I get another brain injury?' For many months, events would be sabotaged by the demon 'What if . . .?' The joy was sucked out of planning pleasurable activities because they would almost always cause upset and as the children were usually behind the fun ideas it was particularly disheartening for them.

But back to the present. Within days of arriving at the O.C.E. Udo's personality seemed to change. This was unexpected as he'd always said that personality tends not to *change* following head injury but aspects of it tend to get exaggerated, so the irritable character might get more short-tempered, the meticulous man even more obsessed with detail. But we were seeing a very different Udo: ignoring others, quite demanding, agitated, with rushed speech and an inability to let topics go. This was not part of his old persona and we were first bemused but then concerned because every day there was less of the man we knew. Imagine our relief when an infection was diagnosed as the cause and a course of antibiotics slowly restored him. This response to infection is not unusual after a stroke. One of the most experienced stroke nurses that we met reminded us that discharged patients are not infrequently referred back to hospital with suspected recurrent stroke only to be diagnosed with a simple infection.

Looking back now, Udo still feels embarrassed by the phase of relentless chatter, which fortunately was limited to only a few weeks. In that time both staff and visitors responded kindly and he was never left feeling shamed by his verbal outpourings, although some staff gently tutored him in the art of reciprocal conversation.

Often the subject of the chatter, which sometimes seemed like free association, was the past because Udo took refuge in the comfort of memories of happier times. In particular he recounted our meeting and the birth of our children, which gave him consolation that his life had not been in vain. He also told and retold stories of his parents' brave endeavours in the Second World War, which reminded him of courage in the face of adversity. The name Kischka means 'guts' in Polish and Udo felt that his parents had lived up to the name: during the war they had survived a salvo of gunfire from British planes, they had leapt from a moving train destined for the Russian death camps and then walked back to Germany. There they had set up a small business from nothing and soon after, Udo's father had even survived being wrongly arrested, imprisoned and sentenced to death by the French. He also recounted how, following bombings, his mother and grandmothers joined with other women searching through rubble. They dug out survivors, found bodies for burial and cleared away debris for rebuilding. They were a familiar sight, known as '*trümmer-frauen*' or 'rubble women' – a brave team creating hope and order from chaos and loss. Udo's recollections weren't intrusive or macabre, the memories of his family's courage and will to survive gave him inspiration and it was good that no one was insensitive enough to silence him because they'd heard it all before.

Despite the kindness of staff and friends it was a hard time and we each sought solace in our own way: the kids watching YouTube; Helen immersed in comforting, escapist DVDs in the early hours of the mornings, while Udo dwelt on his memories or turned to scripture and poetry. One poem in particular inspired him: 'Invictus' by William Ernest Henley. Read it if you can and you'll see why, in such bleak times, it kindled hope with its reference to 'my head is bloody, but unbowed' and 'I am the master of my fate: I am the captain of my soul'. We each need to find something that gives us respite from the bleakness; no one can tolerate distress every waking hour.

With admission to the O.C.E. came a weekday regime of activities. Daily physiotherapy with additional occupational therapy

(OT) and speech therapy gave Udo structure, purpose and most importantly hope. He was energised. Progress was often slight and subtle, but it never went unnoticed. The enthusiastic therapists commented on every positive development and this drove Udo on. After a week, very slight activity was noted in the left hip. Helen heard that this was slight and assumed that it was 'nothing to get excited about', but the never-say-never physiotherapist set us straight: 'No: be excited, be very excited,' because now there was something for the team to work with. Helen and the kids saw little in the way of change, but they were always reassured by Udo and the professionals that progress was being made.

Intensive rehabilitation really inspired Udo and it was noticeable that his mood flattened at the weekends when therapy was limited or went on hold. We tried to buoy things up by making Saturday the fun family day with DVDs and pizza, but it is hard to re-create a family experience in a hospital room and the weekends dragged him down, which in turn dragged down the whole family.

Although there was 'slight movement in the left hip', Udo could feel nothing. He looked at his left leg and arm: he could see them, but still he could not feel ownership. It was as if that half of his body belonged to someone else and he couldn't imagine being connected to it, let alone imagine moving his limbs. The physiotherapist said that unless he could visualise moving his own left arm and leg, deliberate movement would be impossible. This was another blow to us and a scary prospect for Udo: perhaps he would never walk.

A particularly cruel twist was that, although Udo could not feel positive sensations on the left side, he felt pain and he was now more sensitive to it than he ever was before the stroke. He got no pleasure or sensation from Helen's light touch on his hand, yet a gentle squeeze generated intense pain and a light kiss on the left cheek was now an unpleasant experience. He knew that this made sense because the pain pathways to the brain (preserved in Udo's case) are separate from the pathways for touch, but he still found it very unfair. In addition, lifting his leg in rehab exercises caused severe discomfort in his hip, and he was in constant pain from a shoulder that had slipped from its joint because there was no longer enough muscle strength to keep it in place. His dose of painkillers increased, and this meant that he was often more 'woozy' and more lost to us.

Just as the infections had, pain took its toll on Udo's mental state. The sleep deprivation that came from painful nights and the day-long discomforts seemed to make his thinking more muddled and he would veer from a perceptive man to a person known as 'Ditzy Dad' or even (affectionately) 'Muppet'. In this state of mind, he would think that he'd be home in a week, walking in two. He remembered that some patients had been helicoptered to and from the local John Radcliffe Hospital and now he hoped to helicopter to the airport in time for his sister's birthday in Heidelberg in a couple of weeks' time. Once rested and thinking clearly again, Udo was very aware that it was by no means certain that he'd walk again and that his ideas about visiting Germany were grossly unrealistic. This realisation subdued his mood and triggered the embarrassment that was becoming a very familiar feeling.

Staff reassured us with the phrase 'it's early days' but we did wonder how long 'early days' could last. After three weeks, there was little visible change and Helen was returning home at a lower point each evening. It was also taking its toll on our daughter, who described herself as 'a thin plank of wood stretched across a void and each day another brick is placed on me'. Yet she still did not want to talk about her feelings, she simply wanted to disappear to her bedroom, as did her brother. These were the loneliest weeks, despite the support of good friends and family members.

After a month the hemianopia improved somewhat but the hemi-neglect was still evident and reading or TV viewing remained difficult. With no movement in the left side, an inability to entertain himself and extreme fatigue, Udo spent much time in bed, propped up by an origami nest of pillows that was there to stop him from slipping down and to alleviate the hip pain, shoulder pain and now back pain. Thank goodness for visitors.

Visitors gave Udo the energy to keep going, gave him a lifeline to the outside and company that helped him to feel worthwhile. Visitors reminded him that he was worth spending time with. He was more fortunate than some of the patients because we lived locally and could visit once or twice a day. Similarly, many friends were close by and could easily pop in and virtually every one of the staff members was a friend, so he was surrounded by people who would listen as he recounted those well-rehearsed stories of his family. But as the weeks progressed the conversations became more reciprocal and current affairs and literature were also on his agenda. We will always be grateful for those conversations with visitors. If you are a visitor, never underestimate the difference you make, particularly to the person who has been hospitalised for weeks or months. The joy that Udo gained from the visits far outweighed the fatigue that they caused, and he got a sense of achievement from being able to hold a two-way conversation.

He was also inundated with more cards and well wishes from friends, colleagues and patients – and again they raised his and the family's spirits. It was a bitter-sweet experience, though. The cards, letters and e-mails were full of praise for Udo's skills and sensitivities as a doctor and he was clearly a well-respected and able medic, probably at the peak of his career, with much clinical wisdom behind him and doing a great deal of good by all accounts. How hard, then, to have to face the prospect of losing this. Some are fortunate in reclaiming their former life but at this stage many stroke survivors and their families have to contemplate that there might be no going back.

Amid this early grieving a call from Udo's aunt in Italy gave us strength: 'He will recover. It's in his family's blood, Helen. It's who we are.' Although we had to be realistic we also needed hope and we hung on to the aunt's words, grateful that no one dismissed them as fanciful. We also held on to Udo's reassurances: 'In a rehabilitation unit, recovery is measured not in days, not even in weeks, but in months.'

As time passed, Udo grew more aware of the changes in his behaviour: repeatedly watching familiar video clips, recounting the same stories, the emotional lability, the digressions – and his increased awareness made it more difficult for him to bear. The site of his stroke had also given him Parkinsonian symptoms such as the quiet voice, and slowness in moving and thinking. He knew that he was not himself. We tried not to point this out as it simply provoked the all too familiar embarrassment and now a sense of humiliation.

After the first month, however, we did see some physical progress. The rehabilitation was working, and Udo was beginning to combat the complete helplessness that had haunted and scared us so. He began to sit independently and received endless positive comments from staff. He was excited; he felt that he was heading somewhere! Soon after admission, Udo had been regularly placed in a medieval-looking wooden contraption with the distinctive name of the Oswestry Standing Frame. Several physiotherapists would raise him into the frame and secure him with lambskin support straps. At first, he just hung there, wobbling and lacking all muscle tone on the left side, but after about a month there was excitement – there was an indication of thigh movement. Within another two weeks Udo could raise himself slightly within the frame, activating some muscles on the left, and he had begun using a cycling machine that assisted the weak side. He was not yet a multitasker, though: if he cycled he could not chat and if he chatted the cycling ground to a halt.

In parallel we also saw cognitive improvement in that Udo could manage a conversation with more than one person. In the first month a conversation required so much mental effort that it needed to be in a quiet environment with just one person sitting to the right. This gave him the best chance of engaging. At these times his humour, his medical knowledge and wisdom, his logical reasoning were apparent, and Udo was with us again. Add another variable – background noise, a second person, fatigue, for example – and we would lose him. Now this was beginning to change, not dramatically, though, and we frequently witnessed fatigue robbing us of his company, so we had to look for the subtle signs of recovery while bracing ourselves for the many setbacks. This was still the case months later and it is arduous always searching for the crumbs of progress but keeping the daily log helped to keep Udo's development in perspective.

Nonetheless, by the second month following the stroke, Udo's fortitude slipped and one afternoon alone with Helen he spoke of the cost to a man's dignity when he is so dependent on others for the most basic of functions. It was much worse for him, of course, as his carers were also colleagues and some were friends. Then a nurse entered his room, the brave face was restored, and we heard no more of this. Helen now knew what Udo was suffering beneath his stoical surface. Until that afternoon even she thought that he was reasonably comfortable with the situation, perhaps not fully aware of his limitations. It was dreadful to realise that she, his wife, had not been sensitive to his private suffering – and he was suffering. The demands of her own emotional multitasking coupled with Udo's stoicism meant that Helen, quite understandably, hadn't picked up on this and he had borne the distress alone.

Much later, when he was able to reflect on this time, he described it as far more shocking and horrific than he had ever imagined it could be. He found the helplessness devastating, the dependence on others shaming, the fears about the future overwhelming and he discovered his lack of ability to move independently was a significant existential threat – his identity was crushed. He knew that he had always striven to be a compassionate doctor, but he wished that he'd appreciated better the anguish of his own patients and had offered more empathic support when he was still practising.

A friend of ours spoke more openly about a particular aspect of his own struggle in the early days following his stroke. Prior to his brain bleed he had enjoyed a healthy life with no previous hospital admissions and he was quite naïve when it came to hospital procedures. So, he was not at all prepared for what he called the Three Cs that had shocked, restricted and shamed him: catheters, constipation and commodes. Ultimately, he had made a good recovery and was living independently within months, but he could still vividly recount his early experiences as an inpatient and the pervasive sense of shame that threatened his well-being and recovery. He recalled constantly worrying that his catheter would leak urine and that he would smell, so his rehabilitation sessions were often postponed or shortened because he feared this. Such worries dominated his days and when he had visitors he could not fully engage and enjoy the attention of family and friends and they felt that he was distant. Taking heavy-duty painkillers, as he had to, and being inactive tends to cause constipation and so he also suffered from the embarrassment of sitting for long times in a shared bathroom, voices outside enquiring after him, aware that someone else might need to use the facilities. On one terrible occasion the door of the bathroom had not been secured and it swung open as a family of strangers passed by and looked in. The shame of this stayed with him and made him nervous about using the bathroom whilst his need of it was very apparent. The necessary laxatives were sometimes over-efficient, and he then became fearful of being too far from a bathroom just in case he had 'an accident'. One weekend his family had planned a modest day out, but it had to be cancelled because he was so nervous that he constantly asked to be wheeled back to his room, 'just in case'. This was made worse for him because he needed to ask staff to transfer him from chair to commode and any transfer at this time was a source of embarrassment because he was aware that the protective pads that he needed showed above his pyjamas. Although this was a brief period in his rehabilitation he still recalls the time with huge discomfort. Fortunately for him, as is so often the case, his body regained its normal functions within a week or so and he became wholly independent again. Some people won't be so lucky. Udo wasn't; he couldn't transfer himself from his wheelchair for months and some patients will be discharged still needing help with this.

We wanted to know what got our friend through these embarrassing and upsetting times. Not unsurprisingly, he said that the times he felt most at ease were when he was with staff members who were discreet and sensitive. He also told us that he held on to the belief that accepting help with the Three Cs was a means to an end, that enduring the shame would pay off. He believed that taking what help and using what aids were available would speed up his rehabilitation. For those who continue to rely on others, it might be helpful to remind oneself of the 'end point' that makes it worth tolerating the discomfort.

Spirits flag at times like these and in order to keep up morale within the family, Helen stressed the positive: *Dad's beginning to feed himself, he's doing so well . . . Dad's getting stronger, I'm sure he's not slumping over so much . . . Gillian said she had a lovely chat with Dad today, she thinks he's getting better.* Not lies, but not a truly balanced picture and our kids suffered because they were so disappointed at the weekend when their father was still immobile, still needing to be swathed in a plastic apron to eat and still drifting off to sleep at the drop of a hat. Quite rightly, Helen was reprimanded: 'Never, never mislead us like that again. I was so excited, and it's been a shock because I thought he'd be much better than he is.'

There was no denying that progress was slow: Udo was still confined to his room, being hoisted and still easily muddled. But by far the worst thing for those who loved him was that, even in this second month, it was still as if we were visiting a person who was Udo but not Udo. This was the children's 'Imposter Dad', a man who had their father's memories, his values, his face, but something was unnervingly amiss. This was not helped by another consequence of the stroke – a generally expressionless face, a Parkinsonian face, 'Dad's poker face'. It seemed as though he enjoyed nothing, felt nothing and the efforts of the kids to please him fell on stony ground.

In fact, he was truly enjoying their company, their choice of DVDs, their gifts of chocolate, it just didn't show in his expression. Inside he was beaming, but outside nothing.

We also noted some very curious behaviours in Udo, which were as intriguing as they were disconcerting. Activities happening on the left side were still not really noted by Udo at this stage (although there was some improvement over time). We've already described that a person could bid farewell and leave from his left side and as far as Udo was concerned they were still in the room, but if they said their goodbye on his right-hand side he was quite aware that they had gone. Another oddity was that a sound from the left (like a knock on the door) was 'heard' but not attended to – it was simply background noise whereas a knock on the door from the right-hand side was immediately perceived as a welcome noise heralding a visitor and Udo would look up. The same applied to conversation – words spoken on Udo's right-hand side would be remembered but were likely to be forgotten if they were spoken on his left side. Such is hemi-neglect.

The lack of awareness of his own left limbs also contributed to strange experiences and optical illusions. Udo sometimes couldn't distinguish his own arm or leg from that of a nearby person, so he once thought that he was raising his left arm only to be disappointed that it was the arm of the physiotherapist that was moving. He also mistook a long cushion on the floor for his own 'dismembered' arm – quite a shock. Much later, when he had returned home and he had some movement in his arm, he raised it to the light switch and 'saw' his hand become the light switch itself. It was as if it melded with his hand. Udo was able to understand this as '*a faulty connection in the parieto-occipital cortex resulting in the incoming visual and sensory information not being integrated accurately as they would be in a healthy brain*'. As a neurologist he was curious about this but without his specialist knowledge he might have been fearful for his sanity at that moment.

Another bizarre change was in Udo's taste and smell. He could no longer drink fruit juice because within a day it tasted 'too alcoholic'; could no longer eat fish because it tasted 'too fishy'; couldn't bear the 'smell' of the oxygen he had to inhale during an illness. It seems a minor issue given the enormity of the stroke, but it was frustrating – no more pleasurable and refreshing fruit drinks or sushi and the frequent irritation of bad odours that no one else smells. This was yet another thing to be tolerated, along with the chronic pain, the helplessness and the sleep-broken nights. And his sense of pain had changed; it wasn't just that he now had heightened sensitivity, Udo had begun to experience any discomfort as pain. So simply feeling cold or hot was painful throughout his entire body and a chilly night could cause him full-body pain, sleeplessness and general exhaustion. Udo had heard his own patients talk about the difficulties of coping with pain, but he only now knew how disabling this was and that it was not something that was easily addressed by prescribing more painkillers. The painkillers helped but he also had to learn to tolerate pain, to accept and move through it, a skill that he developed with the help of his wise physiotherapist.

Sadly, the setbacks continued, each one emotionally crippling. Yet again we felt we were losing 'Udo', who had become more frail, sleepy and repetitive. He began ringing home in the early hours of the morning to describe his extreme pain, but he would then drop the phone, so we couldn't hold a conversation. His voice had diminished to a whisper, so the chance of a conversation was actually slight anyway. He began drifting off into sleep more frequently and most shocking was seeing him sleep through his first team review meeting. This was a significant planning meeting, a multi-disciplinary gathering to identify realistic goals for treatments and to plan accordingly. This Goal Planning Approach had been pioneered by Udo's colleagues in Oxford many years ago and it is now well established that systematic target setting is very relevant to recovery. Udo knew this, and he had been looking forward to being part of the meeting, seeing it as a vital next step in his rehabilitation, but now he simply could not stay awake. So, it went on around him. Staff spoke on his behalf and Helen took notes in her log book, trying to make the best of the opportunity while he slept and slumped in his wheelchair.

A chest infection was setting in. Another course of antibiotics was prescribed, but this time they didn't work, and his condition worsened although his medical care was excellent, and we marvelled at the prowess of this rehabilitation team. The consultant ordered almost daily chest X-rays and the staff paid very close attention to their patient, but Udo still seemed to be fading by the day. We were worried that we might lose him to pneumonia – it's not unheard of. It was all a bit much and two months after the stroke, for the first time Helen sobbed, properly sobbed.

Eventually Udo did begin to recover from his infection, so we visited *en famille,* waking Dad enough for him to mumble 'Hello', but he then lost the battle to stay awake and slept for hours. The fatigue and sleepiness lasted for days and although we were relieved that the infection had passed we were demoralised by the aftermath. Seven weeks had passed and there was still little *obvious* physical or cognitive improvement and he was still always in pyjamas because he slept so much. More often than not Helen sat by the bedside of a sleeping spouse who was too fatigued to stay awake even though visits meant the world to him. And when Udo did wake, the distractibility was such that random ideas hijacked his attention and conversation was difficult. This was sad and frustrating but again we were reassured – '. . . it's early days . . .' – and it wasn't long before the roller-coaster started to climb again.

At week eight, Helen received a phone call from Udo's main nurse, a wonderful man with whom Udo had worked for years. The big news was that with assistance Udo was able to sit at a sink and wash and shave; it was neither swift nor efficient, but it was happening. The nurse was excited and emotional, and Helen sniffled in the aisle of the supermarket where she took the call, at last daring to hope that we were on a firm upward trajectory. To lift our spirits further Udo's vision was improving as was his appetite, and he was standing with assistance – though not stepping yet. It was time to buy a new daytime wardrobe – soft, washable, elasticated clothes. This might not have been the height of chic but seeing Udo properly dressed gave us all a boost. We wished that we'd done it earlier. There was still very significant paralysis on the left side, hemi-neglect and inattention to deal with; the fatigue remained extreme and the weight loss continued, but we were hopeful again.

One of the hardest aspects post-stroke was, and is, coping with the uncertainty that follows: will he survive? Will he be himself? Will he work again? Will we make it as a family? Will the kids cope? The professionals around us were careful not to give us false hope, which is so very important, but they also seemed conscientious in not dashing our optimism and they always emphasised progress, however slight. Without hope even the most stoical stroke survivor can give up, so getting that balance is crucial. Many seasoned staff members probably saw the signs that progress would be limited following such a large brain bleed, but the majority continued to express cautious and limited optimism about the next step, an approach that kept Udo looking forward to what he might reasonably do rather than dwelling on what he would never manage.

However, this approach, with its moving goalposts, does fuel uncertainty and as time passes the emotional exhaustion of coping takes its toll and it becomes more and more difficult to manage. We all struggled with the early-morning wakening to the what-ifs. *What if there is no functional walking? What if there is no return to work?* Udo kept going by visualising himself with his family post-discharge, just focusing on what he thought was possible in the future. Helen couldn't visualise a positive future but talking things through with friends and family helped her hold on to hope and perspective.

As we've said before, we feel fortunate with our family and friends. Helen had regular visits from good friends and phone calls from a close cousin and a mother who set aside their own worries to offer support. Udo's ninety-three-year-old father phoned from Germany with regular pep-talks and his sister flew over every few weeks to sit by his bedside, feed him German food and to coach him about coping in the future. They devised plans to get him back to his hometown of Heidelberg, and she flooded him with photos and videos of family life back in Germany. Not everyone has such a proactive set of relatives and friends and taking advantage of the therapy offered in the rehabilitation unit or finding community support networks might help others through the bleak times.

Udo for years had worked with Headway Oxfordshire (HWO), the local arm of a national charity that supports head injury victims, and so it was inevitable that after discharge we contacted our local branch, but some stroke victims (patient or family member) might benefit from getting in touch with support networks earlier than this. Organisations like HWO can offer psychological support and practical help even before hospital discharge. Establishing support can fall to the bottom of the to-do list when there seems to be no time between visits, holding the family together, filling in forms, keeping up paid work etc., etc., but we know from decades of psychological research that it will pay off. Since the late 1970s we've known that social support is a very powerful buffer against all kinds of psychological difficulties, and just turning to one person for support can do the trick.

Support from others helped us in dealing with the mass of paperwork and administrative tasks that faced us and which will face anyone whose partner is hospitalised following a stroke: ringing employers, getting sick notes, picking up letters and phone calls from colleagues, identifying unfinished business and trying to tie up loose ends, responding to the taxman who has decided that now is the time for an audit – talk about random events clustering! And it all adds to the stress and the sleepless nights, but wise words and advice from others can make a difference. At the height of Helen's stress about the tax audit, an accountant reviewed the situation and simply said: 'Don't fret.' Those two words from an expert instantly meant a better night's sleep.

Helen had taken the decision to keep all this 'admin' from Udo, to let him focus on his recovery without the concerns of bills and the red tape of HMRC or the Department of Work and Pensions. This was a well-intended but disrespectful decision. Udo had lost so much already, stripping him completely of his role in the family was harsh and with hindsight keeping him more involved might have bolstered his rapidly diminishing self-esteem.

Time passed, and we entered the third month: for most patients in the O.C.E. three months is the total length of their stay, but we were losing hope that Udo would be discharged in January. He was not looking strong and able enough to come home.

When mother and daughter visited, Udo was often pale from sleep loss. The shoulder pain was so extreme during the night that Udo imagined that his arm had been ripped from the socket and now his own severed limb lay across his body. Having no awareness of his left arm meant that it was experienced as unattached to his body, hence the power of the scenario in the early hours of the morning. The painkillers helped, but not enough, and Udo was growing afraid of sleeping at night because of the pain and the nightmares. To make it all worse, the much-needed painkillers then made him groggy during the day.

However, we had an early Xmas present: on day sixty-five we got a message from the physiotherapist: 'The gluts are active!' There was some voluntary movement in the left leg, the gluteus maximus muscles were working and on day sixty-six, Udo stood and stepped. With the aid of an inflatable leg splint to prevent the left knee from collapsing, a euphoric Udo took his first steps and wept. These steps were not yet what is called 'functional' (and we have to admit that they certainly were not elegant) and there were no promises that they ever would lead to independent walking, but the physiotherapists did promise to keep working on it. There was, however, the ongoing problem of Udo not being able to feel attached to his left limbs and without that ability he might not succeed in imagining the stepping movement. Therefore, there was good and bad news, roller-coaster news. Nonetheless, another milestone had been reached and we were again hopeful but uncertain.

Udo had always told his patients that recovery from stroke is a slow and often subtle process; that it's not like in the films when someone wakes up one morning and suddenly they can move their fingers. Udo woke up on day sixty-eight and moved his fingers. It was a very slight movement but one that the physiotherapists could work with. Two days later he squeezed his daughter's hand.

He was also reading again now that his sight had improved. He was using memory tricks – mnemonics – to remember the story plots and characters. His face was getting more symmetrical –although he still had his 'poker face' (and two years on still does). We had made a few videos over the weeks and these really helped us to see this progress in his body strength, movement and facial symmetry.

Heartened by his recent achievements Udo was now working hard towards not needing a hoist to transfer from bed to chair and he was becoming more optimistic that this and other goals were achievable: overly optimistic, in fact. It was mid-December and he began again to talk about going to Heidelberg for Christmas. Despite the recent achievements we all knew that it was impossible; Udo knew that it was impossible and yet he persisted in his hope that he could travel to Germany. He was surrounded by reminders of his disability and limitations, yet the wish was so strong that some part of him saw it as a possibility. This lack of insight in the weeks following brain injury was something that Professor Kischka had often witnessed in his patients – but he couldn't see it in himself.

Suddenly Christmas was upon us and it was the saddest time. As usual the staff was wonderful: they created as festive an atmosphere as possible for all the patients and for three days we were allowed sole use of the O.C.E.'s self-contained practice flat (the unit used to help patients regain their independence during the week) so that we could try to create a more festive experience. But for Udo, Christmas had always happened in Heidelberg. There, the traditions of his childhood were preserved: the Christmas market, illuminated ice-skaters in the shadow of the castle, singing 'Silent Night' around the family's candlelit Christmas tree. Right up until the last moment he'd hoped to find the strength to go but that wasn't to be and on Christmas Eve it was as if the disappointment rendered him unusually weak, muddled and preoccupied. He can barely recall that day.

Helen and the kids had decorated the hospital flat and planned three days of entertainment. But Udo was out of it: he didn't eat, and he repeatedly asked to go back to his hospital room to rest. We spent very little time together. So, when we'd stayed long enough to call it a decent attempt at celebrating, we packed up the unwatched DVDs, threw away the Christmas food, delivered Udo back to his hospital bed and climbed into the car. Little was said but our reserved girl who had not yet cried began to sniff, then she wept inconsolably for the duration of the journey home. There, miserable children disappeared into their own rooms, Helen opened a bottle and we all felt very, very lonely. Our family, despite our best efforts and despite the best support from staff, family and friends, was profoundly fragmented, exhausted and unhappy.

Christmas highlighted our plight rather than gave us respite.

This so-called festive period was made more difficult because, by necessity, the usually full rehabilitation programme was dramatically reduced, and we realised just how psychologically and physiologically motivating it had been. It's Psychology 101 really – physical activity and positive reinforcement are cheering and motivating. Udo literally counted the days until his activities began again.

Things went from bad to worse. The roof of our home started leaking badly and the day after Boxing Day, mother and daughter were bed-bound with chest infections that turned into pneumonia. With buckets strategically placed to catch the rain, we welcomed in the New Year from our sick beds and embraced the numbing effect of the illness and the time out that it offered.

By January 2017, three months were up but Udo needed to stay at the O.C.E. The 'early days' were over.

4

The Long Haul of Rehabilitation: 'One More Whale Song and I'm Out of Here'

Most patients stay at the O.C.E. for three months, some for as long as six. Very, very few stay longer. Udo was an inpatient for nine months. That's a long time to be confined to a hospital room with only a few outings and a repetitive regime. It demands a great deal of patience and tolerance all round. A fellow long-term patient showed the strain of a lengthy stay when he shared his frustration with the relaxation class: 'One more whale song and I'm out of here.'

Three months following the stroke we had seen some progress, but nothing like that experienced by our friend who was home by this time and back at his solicitor's job at six months. Nor was Udo's progress like that experienced by Robert McCrum, the literary editor who chronicled his recovery in his book *My Year Off*: he was home within weeks. Nor was Udo's recovery as speedy as the television presenter Andrew Marr's: he was back in his BBC interviewer's chair after nine months.

Discussing recovery and reading accounts can be helpful in the process of rehabilitation. We certainly absorbed what we could with enthusiasm and hope, yet it is important not to use others as yardsticks for recovery because disappointment can follow. Everyone is different, and this will influence recovery: Udo's stroke was large, and he was in his sixties. He wasn't going to have the same outcome as these younger men. Again, the challenge is in finding the balance between being inspired by fellow sufferers (and survivors) whilst not expecting just the same outcome.

Reviewing others' accounts can urge us on, though. Certainly, Andrew Marr's unsentimental determination will speak to many and help them find fortitude. Robert McCrum's honest observations will ring true for others and offer exquisite insights. Talking with our friend and his family was encouraging, particularly when they repeated what they called 'the wise words of Professor Kischka', words they'd heard three years earlier. They recalled Udo telling them that every recovery is different, that brain plasticity is such that the brain never really stops recovering, but different brains of different ages with different degrees of damage recover at different rates and to different degrees. However, the most inspiring aspect of our talks was their account of the positive changes since the stroke. They had found that in some ways life was now better.

It is easy to focus on loss – and for many stroke survivors the loss is enormous – and teasing out the gains is challenging, particularly once our mood has begun to drop and exhaustion has taken firm hold. So, what were we learning as we entered the long haul of rehabilitation? Apologies for the cliché, but the gift of family and friends is what first comes to mind. Udo, like many parents and spouses who have been dedicated to their work, very quickly regretted family time lost because of his passion for doctoring. His interest in the children and his obvious concern for his wife were now more prominent. This was so very, very important as it helped to bind together a family at risk of coming adrift and provided a sense of teamwork in getting through these dark times. And despite the magnificent work of the rehab team and the wonderful support of friends, these were still dark times.

Discovering genuine caring, bonds that go beyond convenience and fun, was another gift of the stroke. The almost daily texts from Heidelberg; the regular phone calls from family and friends; the kind teachers who kept a watchful eye on our

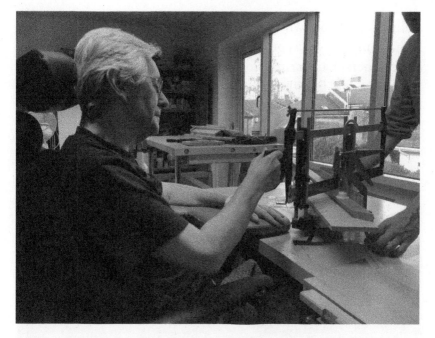

Rehabilitation in the workshop several months after the stroke,
still unable to sit without support

children; the people who came by our home to offer support; the
cohort of friends who turned up regularly to sit with Udo, asking
little in return, which was just as well because he was so often
snoozing. We knew our friends were 'good people', but we had no
idea that there was such kindness amongst them. Months dragged
on but still they turned up with poems and pictures and tempting
foods for Udo and most importantly they bothered to give him
their time. And it was this that helped him regain lost confidence
in himself and to keep a vital connection to the outside world when
his own world had been reduced to a hospital ward for the best part
of the year. Months later, after his discharge, Udo still reflected on
the powerful positive effect that friends had on his rehabilitation.

Perhaps Udo was unusual because among his close acquaint-
ances were some members of staff and he developed a deeper
relationship with so many of them. His unfortunate predicament
meant that he was able to experience first-hand the professional

skills of colleagues who were also friends and among those whom he had only known as professionals he now frequently discovered a more personal, caring side that enhanced his appreciation of them. He did feel that in some ways his life was richer now because of these relationships.

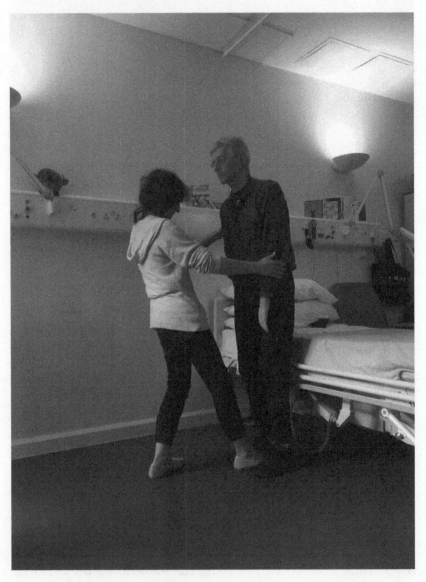

Helen helps an unsecure Udo stand: things are looking up

And by now there were changes to hearten us, for example a graduation from the super-supportive, super-padded wheelchair to a regular wheelchair because Udo's torso was getting stronger. Seeing him sitting without excessive support was thrilling – 'He's looking like Dad again.' This return to a familiar-looking Udo was heightened by his walking using parallel bars and transferring from bed to wheelchair without a hoist. To make things even better, one of our friends commented: 'Udo's personality is gathering strength,' and by four months the clinical psychologist, who already knew him well, declared: 'Udo is back in the room.'

However, fatigue remained a powerful foe. It very quickly stole him away, leaving only a trace of his personality. It left a whispering man who kept his head turned to the right, who didn't engage in conversation, and who gazed into the middle distance. The degree to which Udo's head twisted to the right became our gauge of his level of fatigue (and still is). Sometimes fatigue kicked in just because it had been a long day or because a therapy session had been taxing or perhaps a conversation had run on longer than half an hour, but frequently it was caused by yet another infection. Islands of wit and wisdom were so often unsustainable because of the fatigue and illness.

Although there were times of real clarity in his thinking, we sometimes still struggled in conversation. This was because of a post-stroke tendency to get distracted and to lose the thread of a conversation coupled with a new quality, that of being very insistent and very repetitive. This is all absolutely typical when the frontal lobes of the brain aren't working properly. In Udo's case the lobes themselves were not damaged but the connections to them were, so the wiring was sometimes off. If the frontal lobes aren't properly engaged then it's difficult both to keep focus and to let things go, and this is a bit of a disaster when it comes to chatting. Udo would keep going over the same things again and again, even if we pointed out that he'd now digressed or in fact was wrong in his claims. He wasn't being bloody-minded, though, it was more a compulsion – he just couldn't let go even when he wanted to. As you can imagine, this often created frustration and irritation all round. The good news, at least for us, is that this has improved and keeps improving.

Three months is a tangible amount of time and one expects to be moving on. For Udo this meant that his thoughts turned to work. Being a doctor was not just what he was but who he was, and he could not imagine a life without his work. So began the phase of worrying about resuming his professional role. Increasingly retirement was being talked of and although this was constructive it was perhaps too soon as it raised his anxiety and distress. However, it also increased his drive to work hard in his rehabilitation.

Three or so months is also a long time to be limited to an inpatient unit and it is particularly hard to witness other patients being discharged, more often than not walking out of the unit on their own two legs. Although he hid it from staff and family, Udo was envious. He was perplexed, too. He was working hard, staff told him he was making good progress, doing better than predicted, so why wasn't he ready for discharge? Why wasn't he walking around the unit? Looking back, he should have known better; Professor Kischka would have told him that the size of his stroke would hold him back and make recovery slow. But at that time, he could not have heard these words because he was not yet ready to give up the memory of the life he had lost and hoped to regain. And if he had given up hope, he might have lost his determination to engage so fully in his rehabilitation.

So, even at this advanced stage in his stroke recovery there were still many things that Udo could no longer do and sometimes we, his family, fell into the trap of being critical, as if it was his fault that he'd forgotten something or muddled something or if he couldn't get his sweater on or was over-optimistic. Being blamed for your unwanted problems or overzealous hope can only make things worse. Thank goodness for the patience of the staff members who coaxed and encouraged, who listened and gently re-orientated. We watched and wished that we could muster such gentle acceptance but for a wife or for a child it's frightening to see the person who had been the mainstay of the family so fragile; it upset us, and we sometimes didn't behave in the best way possible.

As time passed, Udo grew more 'psychologically with it' and as he did he was able to recall more of his neuro-rehabilitation experiences as a doctor. Our memories are very much coloured by our current state of mind and Udo was quietly but constantly anxious. Unfortunately, this meant that his recollections were biased accordingly, and he began to recall the patients who didn't make it; those who'd had another stroke, those who'd remained confined to a wheelchair or who didn't get home. This worried him, but he kept his fears to himself because he wanted to protect his family. For similar reasons he also kept his grief to himself but sometimes it showed. One afternoon the hospital transport that was taking him to the dentist was caught up in a traffic jam outside a large guitar store. He said nothing, but a tear trickled down his face. Since boyhood, he'd played the guitar and he knew that he would not know that pleasure again. So often now he felt certain that 'I've lost this – and I've lost it for life'. We might all face this stark reality eventually but following a stroke the limitations can be shockingly abrupt and absolute. There were so many things that were out of his control and no amount of wishing or rehabilitation would help him realise some of his hopes. Little by little, he and our family began to understand and adjust to our new reality.

By now Udo was involved in research trials: hemi-neglect, sleep, community stroke recovery, some of which he'd been involved in setting up. He was pleased to contribute to something useful but sad that he was a subject now rather than the researcher or even the 'healthy control'. This seemed like another reminder of the world that he'd lost, but if he could just wait a few months he would discover that some bleak thoughts are premature . . .

Christmas, birthdays, wedding anniversary and eventually Easter all passed while we were an O.C.E. family. This was eased by two things: first, the kids were tremendously undemanding, content with low-key events, asking for little beyond pizza and cake. Second, we were given weekend access to the practice flat within the O.C.E. It was a 1980s holiday camp of a place, but it was a gift. Once a week, instead of perching on a hospital bed, we sat on chairs and sofas next to Udo; we watched DVDs and episodes of *Doctor Who* while eating pizza; there was carpet underfoot instead of hospital linoleum and depending on the occasion there might also be birthday balloons or festive bunting. This is where we first laughed together as a family watching the antics of the *Top Gear* team and where we could spend time with Udo's sister from Germany, his cousin from the US and dear friends from Sweden. Over the weeks and months following the stroke we had become a fragmented family of four individuals but the flat enabled us to feel unified for a few hours. We often said how constructive it might be if more couples and families had access to similar facilities during weekend visits.

Udo was slowly, slowly getting more mobile but at a price because he now had left hip pain when he stood and when he walked. This was probably because of muscle wastage combined with a bit of osteoarthritis. He became very impatient because this slowed down his progress. As a neuro-rehabilitation specialist he had been perplexed by his patients' predominant desire to walk; it was often their only goal. He couldn't understand why they focused so keenly on walking when rehabilitation can offer so much more, but now he was just as single-minded as his patients had been and anything that held up his walking practice frustrated him. Although he was increasingly aware of the limitations of his left arm (he could not cut food or dress himself), improving his arm and hand movement was always less pressing than walking.

Helen quizzed him about this, because it was particularly hard for her to understand why he would prioritise mobility over recovering his cognitive abilities, abilities that she thought would make him feel more like his old self. He explained that he now realised that standing and moving were fundamental to his sense of self – for the first time he appreciated that being unable to take a few independent steps when necessary, or to spontaneously stand, or to look visitors in the eye all robbed him of his sense of who he was. No wonder he, and so many of his patients before him, wanted to stand and walk and how hard it must be for those who never achieve this.

He was sometimes frustrated because he simply wanted to go to the gym and practise walking, walking, walking and instead his precious gym time was focused on learning to balance, or just on working through pain or visualising his left side. Then, a week or so later, he would have a wonderful session when he would practise walking and realise how all these earlier elements of physiotherapy cleverly came together, falling into place like pieces of a puzzle. Then the preliminary work made sense and made him a better walker. As his very wise physiotherapist pointed out, he wasn't just learning to propel himself forward but to position himself safely, to be precise in his footfall, protecting his joints from pain. He was learning skills for life and if he didn't learn to walk properly he could be setting himself up with problems for life.

At twenty-two weeks, that's five months after the stroke, our daughter visited the hospital to witness her dad walk using just a quad stick and to watch him transfer himself from a wheelchair to the car. There was excitement and anticipation, but it was not a good day – Udo struggled, wobbled and fell back into the wheelchair. He felt clumsy and insecure again and he was deeply disappointed. The previous physiotherapy sessions had gone so much better. A few minutes later he returned to the familiar parallel bars in the gym and 'nailed it', as our kids would say. He walked well, supported by a handrail on either side, and his teenage girl sniffled a few tears of joy. However, we had noticed that Udo's performance tended to deteriorate when family members came to watch. The simple fact was we made him nervous and distracted him, and because his mobility was so fragile, this frequently impaired his performance. We decided that it was for the best if we didn't come to watch any more. We did ask others to make brief videos of his physical progress and this has proved invaluable because we have a visual record of his improvement over time. Although progress has been slow and even now his stamina is not great, we can look back over the films and see an increasing precision and elegance in his gait.

Our spectating days were over, but we hoped that Udo's physical recovery would benefit. Not for the first or last time our thinking was naïve; Udo could now concentrate better in the gym and he began to do more, but there was a physical/psychological pay-off. Beyond a certain point, the more gym work and walking practice he did, the more muddled and sleepy he became and the less interested he was in his visitors. His sister had once again travelled all the way from Heidelberg only to discover a rather detached brother. 'He isn't interested in me today,' she told us when we joined her at the hospital. He wasn't *able* to be interested in anyone: at this point in recovery it was too much to ask of him to work hard physically and then perform socially. Unfortunately for us, his drive to walk was so great that time after time he exhausted himself in the gym and then slept or seemed dazed during visits. This was disappointing for Helen, the kids and anyone else who had taken time to see him but maybe it was worth it.

Almost six months after the stroke, there was good news from the physiotherapists. For weeks since the first stand and leg movement we'd been told: '. . . can't promise that Udo will be able to take functional steps'. Now we heard: 'This is proper walking, Udo!' In fact, his physiotherapist was confident that he'd walk with a stick. To add to our delight, Udo's attention seemed to be improving, the multitasking was getting a bit easier, although walking and talking in English would elude him for some time. He could, however, walk and chat in German and Italian (his first and second languages) and he had the opportunity because the staff at the O.C.E. was such an international bunch.

In parallel with the physiotherapists' work on walking, the occupational therapists had been helping Udo regain the use of his left arm and hand. They spent time massaging his swollen hand and introduced him to a wide range of exercises including visualisations of everyday activities, repetitive arm movements, picking up objects. One task was called the 'mirror box' and Udo was very sceptical of it. It comprised a tunnel of a box with a mirrored exterior. The idea was that the paralysed arm went into the tunnel and then the working limb was reflected in the mirror so that, when the functioning arm moved, it created the illusion that both were working, and the brain would be tricked into thinking that the paralysed arm worked. This would then stimulate the part of the brain that would usually move the weak limb.

Udo was very averse to this therapy, convinced that his neurologist's brain could not be tricked, and for some weeks he just pushed it aside. Fortunately, the occupational therapists weren't nearly so easily pushed aside. They persisted and then, after only a few sessions of using the mirror box, the left hand really did start to perform movements in tandem with his right. This kick-started a neurological process and the active movements in his left hand and arm began improving. The optical illusion was far more powerful than his professional scepticism. Thank goodness.

The occupational therapist also worked on Udo's intellectual functioning in collaboration with the clinical neuropsychologists and he was encouraged to review academic papers, although his focus remained physical improvement. Looking back, it's not even clear that Udo was aware of his cognitive limitations even though he was acutely aware of his physical restrictions. Helen remained disappointed about this because she wanted him to regain his concentration and other cognitive abilities so that she could resume proper conversations and feel that her help-mate and companion had returned. This difference in opinion persisted right up until discharge, but Udo was pretty immovable on this one.

Looking back, his prioritisation of walking made sense psychologically. In the 1940s Abraham Maslow came up with a theory of what motivates people. It's called 'Maslow's hierarchy of needs'. It states that humans are initially motivated to satisfy their *physiological* needs and only then do they look to the next stage, *safety*, and only when they feel safe are they motivated to achieve a sense of *belonging*, and only then do they seek *esteem* from others and for themselves, and finally humans strive for what he called *self-actualisation*, which is a very sophisticated state of achieving self-fulfilment and personal growth. Udo could not yet stand and walk, and he felt afraid most of the time, so of course he was going to be motivated to focus on his physiological needs and until they were met he would be poorly motivated to do much else. Helen, however, wanted to see self-actualisation, she wanted Udo to be striving for his full psychological potential but, as Abraham Maslow could have told her, this was premature. For many months she would have to tolerate the frustration of not seeing Udo strive for the same goal that she held for him.

It was now spring, and as the weather improved Helen could wheel her husband to the local shops and dine with him in a nearby café in the middle of the day. On the one hand it cheered us to get out of the O.C.E. and the four walls of the hospital room, but we soon learnt the difficulties of a middle-aged wife managing a grown man in a wheelchair. The slightest incline felt like Everest, our movements were determined by the availability of dropped kerbs and the quality of the surface of the pavement; choices of café or restaurant were limited by door width and steps, and we discovered that Udo felt painfully self-conscious. In the real world of ambulant people, he felt disabled. People older than us were walking freely, even hand in hand, and Udo felt that life as he knew it was over because this was lost to us and he couldn't imagine regaining it. After years of encouraging his patients to get out and about in a wheelchair, Udo discovered that far from being cheered by this he felt hopeless and embarrassed – not ashamed because there was nothing to be ashamed of, but he hated being seen so helpless and no longer the professional that he had been. On these outings Udo just wanted to return to the hospital and get back to the gym. He'd been confronted by his inability to walk and he wanted to practise walking again and again.

By six months, we heard fewer reassuring noises from staff, but Udo seemed to be gaining some stamina both physically and mentally. He began to show off his party pieces to friends

– standing and walking a few steps with a quad stick, conversing while cycling, moving his fingers – albeit in a rather random fashion. He was proud yet embarrassed because it felt so little to show for months of intense rehabilitation. This was still far from what Udo had hoped to achieve and time was running out.

Despite obvious progress, there had been no home visits yet. The problem was our home – a tall terraced house with a flight of steps front and back. Creating disabled access had to be negotiated with the city conservation office and this was a protracted and frustrating procedure that dragged on for weeks and weeks. Until we had permission to install a small temporary chair lift over four steps at the back of the house, we simply could not get Udo into his home and that meant that he could not visit. We were tormented by the worry that we wouldn't secure permission in time for discharge. He would then have to go to a care home. And if permission was refused, an entire family would have to sell up and move at a time when they were least emotionally resourced to do so. As if any family in crisis needs to be faced with these difficulties too.

Thus, it was months before he could visit his own home, and when he did it was not because we had finally gained permission to install a small chair lift, but because Udo climbed stairs. Members of the physiotherapy department had been honest with him and told him that he didn't have the muscular strength to tackle stairs, but angered by the city conservation office and driven to some extent by fear, on day 202, Udo climbed up and down four practice steps. Three weeks later, in early May, he climbed the steps into his own home, pottered across the kitchen and sat in a real chair and said: 'Today I feel like a man with two legs.'

After his successful ascent, which was despite the reservations of staff, Udo had told a friend of his achievement. 'That's like the bumble bee,' said our friend. 'It's aerodynamically unfit to fly but it doesn't know this, so it just flies.' For a while Udo was known as 'The Bumble Bee'. But his achievement wasn't simply an adrenalin-fuelled miracle; he had been able to exceed his physical limitations because parts of his body other than his left leg were compensating for the weakness in his paralysed limb. His stronger right side was holding him, moving him forward, pulling the weak side upward and along, and with practice it got better.

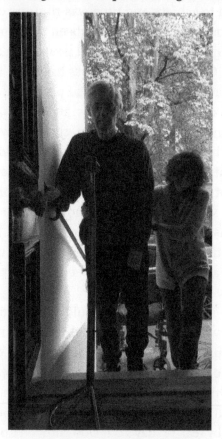

The bumble bee returns home

Things seemed to be coming together at last and the graded return home had begun. Quite rightly, returning home was to be introduced in stages, beginning with an afternoon, then a day, then an overnight stay, then a weekend with the family. We'd been excited about home visits and had expectations that we would regain a sense of family and optimism. But after more than seven months away, home life was not as perfect as we'd hoped. Udo had his O.C.E. routines and Helen and the kids their no-Udo routines and there was awkwardness and disappointment.

The transport and transition involved in a visit was exhausting and more often than not Udo ended up sleeping during the visits and waking just in time to return to the unit. Nonetheless, he was extremely happy to be home and it confirmed to him that this was his main priority, but he was growing increasingly worried how helpless and vulnerable he was. At last, his concerns broadened from his ability to walk to his ability to care for himself and he began to put more energy into his remaining OT rehabilitation sessions where he was learning to dress. Now he was worried that his self-care would still be poor on discharge and that he would have to sacrifice a good deal of independence.

But help was at hand, the community OT (working in harmony with the O.C.E. OTs and physiotherapists) was determined to get Udo in the shower, using the bathroom, making lunch and working on his laptop by whatever means the community services could provide. For weeks we had deliveries of seat raises, stools, side tables, grab handles, all of which were trialled at home. We kept those that helped and eventually we had a little collection of aids that did make a difference thanks to the determination of a rehabilitation team that could think in 4D, projecting into the future what we might need in our home. They were fantastic and again we were reminded of the high quality of staff in the NHS and social services. Do be aware just how many of these aids are provided by the NHS – don't do as we did and start buying them. We soon discovered that we'd spent an unnecessary amount on minor house adaptations because we'd assumed that this was wholly our responsibility.

By now we were spending more time as a family but as we did, we noticed more oddities that were unsettling. Helen got upset because there were occasions when Udo not only forgot things, but he seemed to recall things that hadn't happened. Nothing so huge that you'd consider them significant false memories, but little things such as snippets of conversation that she was sure hadn't taken place or decisions that were quickly forgotten.

Looking back this most often happened when a conversation had been to Udo's left side and we now appreciate that his hemi-neglect interfered with his ability to process and recall what came from that side.

'Udo, have you telephoned your dad? You said you would.'

[Pause] 'No, you told me to wait.'

'I didn't. I thought that we'd agreed that you'd do it this after-noon. I did say: "In your own time," and then you said you'd get on to it.'

'No, you told me to wait.'

'I didn't, Udo; really I didn't.'

Helen pointing this out left Udo feeling puzzled, attacked and misunderstood and this often became a source of tension. Then one evening a penny dropped and with the satisfaction of having solved a mystery, our neurological Sherlock Holmes, Udo, announced: 'Gestalt is a very real phenomenon and the brain is so good at it.' In a household of psychologists, one might have hoped that we'd have come to this realisation earlier but better late than never.

The term Gestalt was introduced into psychology to describe the process by which our minds bring together pieces of informa-tion and make sense of them even if there are parts missing. There is a very simple diagram that illustrates this:

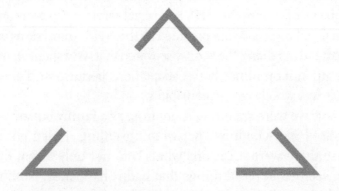

Most of us will immediately 'see' a triangle even though there is no triangle, only three shapes that don't connect. We see the entire

triangle because we rapidly and unconsciously fill in the gaps creating a whole entity from fragments – hence the Gestalt misquotation: 'The whole is greater than the sum of its parts.'* It's a very vital mental ability that increases our information processing speed and it usually makes us much more efficient because we are not constantly trying to compensate for little bits of missing information. For example, if we see our GP sitting behind her desk we don't anguish over her missing legs, we have an automatic awareness that they are there. If a cow walks behind a slender tree and we can no longer see its middle, we fill in the gap and still perceive an entire animal.

Udo now realised that he tended to miss some information coming from his left side because of his hemi-neglect, thus he had more than the average number of gaps. His brain then did what human brains have been doing for generations – it filled in the gaps, but in doing so it could introduce things that hadn't taken place. In his case the amount of 'filler information' might be more than usual and as a result his recollections of conversations or activities could become a little distorted. Typical of the Gestalt effect, the reconstructed picture felt 'right', just as when we look at the figure above we feel quite confident that we are looking at a triangle. So, Udo did not feel the need to question himself.

In the example above, Udo and Helen had a conversation and Helen heard them come to a decision that he'd contact his father. Udo really had intended to phone his dad, indeed he looked forward to chatting with him, but because the conversation with Helen had been to his left, his recollection of it was not complete and he was also now more distractible since his stroke, so the task got side-lined. Later, when Helen asked him if he'd made the call, it didn't make sense to him that he'd not done something that he'd so wanted to do, and he had no recollection

---

* The correct quotation for the Gestalt phenomenon is: 'The whole is something else than the sum of its parts.'

of making a commitment. It was understandable, however, if he'd been told to hold off ringing his father. Then it made sense. The gap was filled. It felt right. Hence his conviction: 'No, you told me to wait.'

The realisation that Udo was simply experiencing the Gestalt phenomenon was very reassuring: he wasn't going crazy; his brain was simply being over-efficient at times. And as with so many other post-stroke quirks, this has improved over the months.

But all was not plain sailing – remember California Screaming? There was no escape from it, and we were bound for another roller-coaster ride. By mid-May, things were slipping again. Udo's voice was barely a whisper, his attention easily strained, his gaze preferred the right-hand side and fatigue had returned with a vengeance. And so it went on, just weeks before discharge and things were getting worse not better. Udo was losing weight again, he could no longer reliably transfer from wheelchair to ordinary chair because he was too weak, he stumbled more frequently, he slept for hours during the day, he reported feeling 'woozy' and it was harder for him to think straight. Even the muddled late-night calls began again. The consultant called for another brain scan to see if there had been further brain damage, and mercifully there was no evidence of a further stroke. So why this extreme setback? With hindsight there seemed to have been a perfect storm of events.

First, he had been overdoing the physical rehabilitation. He was walking as much as possible, attending two physiotherapy sessions daily and cycling for over an hour before bed, sometimes falling asleep on the machine. The team decided to limit his phys-ical activity, which was wise, but this was not the only culprit.

Medications that lower blood pressure tend to make a person groggy and Udo was still taking blood pressure tablets. By now it was a treatment that had outlived its need, so it was stopped but even this didn't return Udo to a more energetic self because our old adversary the infection was back. This time it was not so swiftly dealt with by antibiotics and it required repeated treat-ments, setting back progress (and optimism) for at least a month.

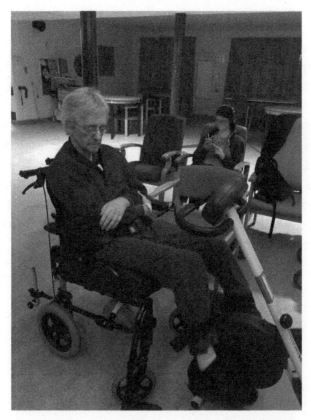

Nearing discharge: exhausted on the cycling machine

At home the drama continued. Just a week before Udo was due home, we discovered that we couldn't install the internal stairlift that we had ordered in anticipation of his return. The fitter walked into the house and announced, 'Well, that's not going to happen,' and sure enough it didn't. The original salesperson had measured up wrongly and this particular company could not actually accommodate our very steep stairs. Finding another supplier took time and we feared that Udo would have to go into a care home after all because he wouldn't have access to a bathroom and bedroom. Luckily the discharge officer was quick-thinking and practical and we were immediately loaned a hospital bed to be put up in the front room close to the downstairs cloakroom. Helen was initially uneasy about this. She recalled as a child visiting poorly relatives who had transferred to a bed in the parlour in their final days, so the thought of Udo lying in the study was disturbing, especially as this was where she had found him nine months earlier. But as with so many things, the anticipation was much more dramatic than the reality; we adjusted really quite quickly, and it simply became our temporary norm.

Leaving the O.C.E. for what turned out be the last time as an inpatient, we wheeled Udo past a mother pushing her newly admitted son in a very heavy-duty wheelchair. He was slumped as Udo used to be and he seemed unable to communicate. Helen so wanted to reassure the mother that this is a miracle hospital, but British reserve got in the way and nothing was said.

5

Re-entering the Real World: 'Plasticity and Tenacity'

The discharge date came and went. Without available care in the community to help with the transition, Udo couldn't leave the rehabilitation unit. The community resources were (and are) so strained that there is a waiting list for community support and without it a patient simply cannot be sent home. It's a necessary safety issue, but one that transformed Udo from inpatient to bed-blocker.

We had prepared for the big day of discharge. Helen had made 'Thank you' cakes for the various departments, each with a sugar figure of a man wearing spectacles and a grey suit (i.e. Udo) but he remained on standby for another couple of weeks. During this time staff did what they could to maintain a meaningful programme but being in limbo was disconcerting and not really productive. Days came and went then, during a routine visit home, we got the call: 'Care in the community is available – there is no need to come back to the O.C.E.' Nine months had passed and at last Udo was discharged. No ceremony, no goodbyes and no cake.

It was more anti-climactic than we'd expected. We'd had a fantasy about the return home. We had imagined that it would come at a time of renewed ability, not lingering disability; that we would know what would come next, but we still didn't; that harmony would reign now that we had learnt to appreciate each other – but it was often far from harmonious. At some point Udo said: 'You were so nice when I was in the hospital, Helen.' This was probably true but as visitors we only had to pull out the stops and hide the fears and frustrations for a few hours – now we had to do this 24/7. Also, Udo was now under scrutiny from us all of the time and we saw new aspects of him. Until now his family had seen little of the befuddled-early-morning or oh-so-tired-at-night Udo or the Udo who was scared now that he no longer had the security of the hospital. It was upsetting to witness these times of muddled thinking or acute distress about falling, or fears about suffering another stroke or the sadness that he had not reached his personal goals (which were in excess of the goals set by the O.C.E.).

It was downright alarming seeing him sleep for hours on end, far more than he had in the hospital. When he did get up it wasn't long before he felt the need to nap again and in total there were very few waking hours. Helen began to worry that Udo had suffered another stroke because she too lived in fear of 'the second stroke', but then, after two weeks of slumber, he awoke. It was as if he'd caught up on nine months of lost and broken sleep in hospital and on the afternoon of his proper waking he returned to us. For the next few weeks Udo slept long and heavily but the 'Rip Van Winkle' phase had passed. Looking back, Udo did wonder if wearing earplugs at night while in hospital would have protected him against developing such a sleep deficit.

Around this time, Helen was reminded of coming home with a new-born: on one's feet all the time ministering, checking that the loved one is still breathing, schedules going awry, even the best laid plans getting hijacked, and as for sleep ... But it was good to have Udo home, caretaking for ourselves and not delegating to others. And Udo was so very obviously happy to be back in the family fold.

Music had always been very important to Udo. Years ago, he'd busked with a lute in Heidelberg, as a student he had composed a rock opera (unpublished) and for a while he was the president of Germany's oldest jazz club. He says – and maybe this is true

– he decided to marry Helen within days of their meeting because she recognised a Thelonious Monk tune that he was humming. So, it was merciful that the right-sided bleed had not robbed him of his ability to enjoy music, and to celebrate Udo's homecoming Helen had planned an outing to a local piano recital. The concert had been carefully chosen to motivate him: the musician was his very, very favourite pianist, András Schiff, according to Udo one of the few musicians who could bring Bach to life. Even so, as the day of the concert approached, it was clear that he would not be able to attend. Disappointingly, nearly ten months after the stroke he still did not have the mental stamina to concentrate for more than an hour and we knew that he would be so exhausted by the transfers between wheelchair and car that he would probably soon be slumped and asleep. Not a good way to communicate his appreciation of Schiff, so we cancelled the outing and Helen made a mental note not to be overambitious. We'd fallen into the trap of thinking that once Udo was home we would be able to resume old social and domestic activities, but this was still a very long time away.

Being back in the real world, back in our home together, high-lighted how different our family life was compared to our pre-stroke existence. Initially we were more aware of the losses than we had been when we were protected from the extent of Udo's disabilities by hospital care and provision. Now we more clearly saw his limitations and realised our own.

Helen and the kids worked particularly hard at maintaining the 'glass half full' mindset. At least Udo had been able to come home rather than having to go to a care home; at least he had the power of speech; at least Helen had a job and an income . . . These 'at least's filled entire days. It was conscious and effortful but necessary to keep from slipping into the trap of dwelling on what we'd lost rather than focusing on what we had. This strategy didn't work so well for Udo who, confronted with new realities now he was home, more and more simply felt the loss: loss of mobility, loss of tiny freedoms, loss of his role as a father, as a help-mate and as a doctor . . . And so the list went on. He hadn't anticipated just how much these losses would threaten his self-concept, but he discovered that his sense of identity was profoundly challenged. His feeling of no longer being the person he had been for sixty years was amplified on outings in the wheelchair when hardly anyone looked him in the eye or spoke with him directly. When friends and colleagues did look at him they nearly always had to look down, which left him feeling pitied and gave him a feeling of no longer being part of this tribe – even if he consciously knew this not to be the case.

With characteristic humour and humanity, the author Terry Pratchett wrote about his experience of dementia in his book, *A Slip of the Keyboard*. Although Udo's brain damage wasn't progressive like Pratchett's, there was much we could relate to in his writings, in particular his feeling of being diminished, which could equally apply to those disabled by a stroke: 'It seems that when you have cancer you are a brave battler against the disease, but when you have Alzheimer's you are an old fart.'

Udo gradually entered a period of grieving that would last for months. We didn't see this as pathological but as a normal response to our new reality and his loss of who he had been.

Before his stroke Udo had advised his patients to focus on what they could still do rather than dwelling on what was no more and to engage in activities that they could manage. He did this with the best intention but when he received the same advice – often from his wife – it wasn't helpful. It was too soon. He needed time to mourn the loss of his previous life and hopes. Much, much later, as his period of grieving eased, he could see more possibilities, but he was able to do this because time had passed and he'd reached his own conclusions, not because his wife had nudged him into optimism.

What did help Udo at this time was reviewing happy and hopeful memories. He may have lost the future that he'd taken for granted but he still had memories that made a difference to him. So, he'd trawl the internet for pictures of Heidelberg, his university graduation, his family holiday spots and his friends. He needed happiness in his life so that he could mentally escape the confines of a semi-paralysed body. To some extent this worked for him, although everyone has to find his or her own way of getting through.

A surprising discovery – surprising because we were both seasoned clinicians and we should have appreciated this – was just how very much a constructive discharge report can help a family to look forward with hope and motivation. For several years before his stroke, Udo had carried out assessments for law firms that arranged rehabilitation for people who had suffered brain injury through accidents. He often had access to their end-of-treatment reports and he recalled that the best long-term rehabilitation plans were frequently built not just on his assessment but on this coupled with information from a discharge plan that recorded what had been beneficial to the patient, where their strengths lay, what resources existed to support the person in the longer term and what might be reasonable goals for the future. When we received Udo's discharge report we were instantly aware of the psychological and practical impact of a constructive, forward-looking document.

If you are able to preview and discuss your report, you might be able to ensure that your abilities are emphasised at least as much as your disabilities and that your prospects and potential are clearly spelt out. A document that captures abilities, strengths and possibilities (rather than one that simply dwells on disability and limitations) can revive hope as well as providing a very productive guide for the community professionals who take on the longer-term care and treatment.

As you might discover, there are many little, cruel aspects of having a stroke: no longer being able to play a much-loved instrument or to enjoy a meal that requires both hands to be working well. For us a niggling cruelty was finding that we were not able to share a bed after all this time of being apart. The shoulder pain that Udo continued to suffer meant that he needed to remain in the single hospital bed in the study. The nine months of lonely nights extended to more than ten months, with trials and trials of mattresses and positioning of pillows. Eventually we discovered the memory-foam-mattress-topper and the precise positioning of pillows that allowed Udo to sleep without too much discomfort and permitted us to share a bed – just that, just sharing a bed because even cuddling caused terrible shoulder and hip pain. But lying parallel we could chat into the wee hours, we could hear each other breathing at night, knowing that we weren't alone. It was a huge step forward; there was hope that we could be a team again. We couldn't hold hands under the covers, though – at least, Helen couldn't hold Udo's left hand. If he wasn't able to see his upper limb he couldn't visualise his hand being held, and any pressure was uncomfortable to the point of being intolerable. His pain threshold had shifted, and it took very little to trigger extreme discomfort. Nonetheless, we were moving forward – after a fashion.

Udo learnt a lot about pain in that first year. That it was an almost twenty-four-hour, every-day-of-the-week experience that kept him awake, held him back, exhausted him both physically and mentally. Pain-relief medications gave him some respite, but it was limited relief and the drugs often made him woozy.

Helen only really began to appreciate his battle with pain when she suffered a bad bout of sciatica. She blamed herself – it was all because of her brush with glamour in her late teens. Back then she'd toured Staffordshire working men's clubs as a hair model and she'd flirted with the Manchester rag trade (less couture-for-celebrity, more mass-production-for-the-marketplace, though). She'd entered the spirit of this glam world, embraced the appropriate accessories and wrecked her back in the process. Twenty-five years later, a neurosurgeon studied scans of her spine, identified the sad slipped discs and declared this a typical 'high heels and heavy handbags' injury.

Well, now her fashion choices were back to haunt her. She was in pain and she could fully empathise with Udo's absolute exhaustion by midday, his decisions to avoid doing things because even tiny movements triggered Taser-like agony, and his taking an age to shift a limb because it required military-level planning to make a movement safe. She also realised why he would become so very annoyed if she said: 'Just reach over for this or that' or 'Just stand up' or 'Just move this way'. The concept of 'just' meaning a simple thing does not exist when you are wracked with pain, or indeed half paralysed. 'Just' fell from the Kischka vocabulary.

Bent with discomfort we were both limited in our mobility and agility, a brace of Richards IIIs tentatively inching our way around the house, incapable of carrying out the most basic domestic chores. We realised how much any couple in our situation relies on the caretaker being well and Helen regretted not keeping up her Pilates and her core strength exercises. Every day she would remind Udo that he must exercise to build the muscle strength to hold his shoulder and hip in place, but she'd side-lined her own fitness regime. Easily done when life seems crammed with other to-dos. In our helpless and hapless state, we were saved by our two teenagers who went on foraging missions to the local super-market – better that than exam revision – and kind neighbours who'd give them lifts to their clubs and classes. We were lucky to have ready access to back-up – do make sure that it is there for you, too.

There were still great ups and downs in this phase of recovery, reasonably 'good' days followed by totally 'bad' ones that took us right back to the frightening early days in the hospital when Udo was known as 'Imposter Dad' or 'Muppet'. The downs related both to Udo's capabilities, which varied enormously from day to day, and to the well-being of our family. In particular, the kids could find the new set-up very hard going. Adjusting to the pres-ence of a father so different from their pre-stroke dad was far from easy. Our daughter articulated some of her difficulties, but her younger brother was silent, and we could only speculate on his distress as we saw him distancing himself. He still hadn't told his teachers about the stroke and from that we guessed that it was hard for him to accept what had happened.

We began to identify the patterns, the predictors or at least correlates of difficult times – not enough sleep, low blood pressure, a dip in mood and it would be a 'bad' day. There were 'good' days too, but progress felt very fragile and Udo was vulnerable and, just as in hospital, he was frequently set back again by infection. The setbacks distressed Helen and she asked Udo how he felt about these great ups and downs. He was rather unfazed by it all and explained that it was no different from his experiences at the O.C.E.; he was now used to this way of being. What was different, he said, was his wife's grumpiness about it all.

We also learnt more about the best and the worst of the public. We soon discovered that the majority of pedestrians didn't make way for a woman pushing a man in a wheelchair, frequently forcing us to the kerb where we felt very vulnerable. This hadn't happened when we'd pushed baby buggies all those years ago and perhaps the difference was that people look into a baby buggy, often with a friendly smile, knowing how to react. In contrast, many people looked away from us and carried on walking as if disability didn't really exist. When face to face with us and forced to converse, very few people spoke to Udo. Even those sitting at the same level as him looked over his head and addressed Helen. Udo had expected this, so it didn't surprise him nearly as much as it upset the rest of the family.

Despite now having the marvellous Blue Badge for parking, we discovered that we were still restricted. One chilly afternoon we visited Christchurch Picture Gallery, which involved a memorably bone-shaking wheelchair ride over cobblestones. Udo had always loved art and it was with great relief that we learnt that his full sight had returned so that he could again enjoy exhibitions and galleries. But it wasn't to be that day: there was no wheelchair access. It's understandable that a historic building might not be granted permission to create access for the disabled, we do understand that, but this was one of very many disappointments that just drag a person down. Now we've learnt to scout things out to avoid discouraging incidents, and in doing so have discovered some terrific Oxford venues that are positively wheelchair welcoming: the Ashmolean Gallery, the Woodstock Museum Café, a new burger bar in the city centre. So, the glass was still half full.

And we had experiences that showed us the best in people, too. Udo had worked as a doctor in West and East Germany, Holland, the US and in 1998 he moved from an exceptionally well-resourced Swiss Rehabilitation clinic to work in the NHS in Oxford. He took a cut in salary, he lost his spacious office and personal assistant, he had to work with limited resources and yet he always said that the move was a gift because NHS workers are beyond compare. He was reminded of this every day of his rehabilitation and no less when the community carers came to his aid following discharge. We rarely saw the same person twice, but they were without exception caring and professional and several were outstanding: cheery despite the hour (which could be early morning or late in the evening) and despite heavy workloads and frustratingly inadequate training for the wide demands of the job. Udo's long compression stockings flummoxed a few and his shoulder support was a constant source of bewilderment – and also of creativity. The most impressive positioning of this contraption was when someone mistakenly fastened it around his waist, strapping in the left arm above the wrist. Udo had slight movement in his fingers so when he now flexed them outwards he did a good impersonation of a penguin. Nonetheless this small army was an absolute boon and we missed them sorely when our allocated six weeks of help was up.

Headway Oxfordshire (HWO) was also marvellous. Our contact person was full of gentle wisdom and assurances about families getting through and she was superb in helping us complete the various forms for disability support. You must apply for your personal independence payments (PIP) as this benefit helps with the extra costs incurred by disability, and they can be substantial.

Headway, like other similar community-based organisations, can provide much needed support and information for the entire family. So do find out where your local support is as early on as possible – even before discharge.

There were other reminders of the best of humanity: finding a dear neighbour clad in wellies and Marigolds cleaning Udo's neglected car; the friends who still popped round and who scouted out venues for us; the gift of a much-valued exercise bike from someone who did not know us well but who was deeply kind; the considerate porters who positioned Udo over a heating vent on the chilly evening of a carol service in Magdalen College chapel; family members who never forgot us; neighbours who sent greetings and even now left food parcels on the doorstep. So good was the cuisine from our neighbours that our son told us that he was 'sad about Dad's stroke, I really am, but you have to admit the food's better now'. You have to know Helen's cooking to realise that we couldn't argue with him on this one.

When the dedicated army of community carers ceased their visits, Helen took on their role. After six weeks there had been progress: Udo was still woozy but, overall, he was more alert during the day, more focused, with an increasingly reliable memory, and this made practical tasks easier. He was able to wriggle the fingers of his left hand and to make a Napoleonic gesture when walking – the left arm was becoming biddable at last and indeed was reasonably adept at holding a deodorant stick or a toothbrush – as long as he could see it. If the object and his left hand were out of sight, then the deodorant or the toothbrush would tumble to the floor.

Preparing for bed was no longer a big deal but dressing in the morning required more input because the shoulder support, the compression stockings and the ankle splint would tax even the most able-bodied. It was around this time that we grew to understand the reality of 'use it or lose it'. Once Udo was able to do something again, something such as putting on his pyjama top or adjusting his sweater, we tumbled into the trap of assuming that he had fully regained the skill and we could now ease up on practice. So, Helen relaxed the rehab and stopped attending to parts of the dressing regime. After all, it was far quicker to substitute a T-shirt for the pyjama top and she could speed things along by taking a lead in dressing Udo. Shockingly, a month later these self-dressing skills had all but disappeared. The stroke had affected the right hemisphere – the seat of spatial ability, an ability needed for dressing – and without repeated rehearsal and practice the skill faded. Helen had probably been wrong, the old skill had not been resurrected – the old ability had been obliterated by the brain bleed and now a new part of the brain was taking over, and in order to do so it needed lots and lots of practice. The good news was that these skills (wherever they now resided in the brain) were revived quite quickly, but they were not as they had been before the stroke. We had to adjust to the fact that Udo's spatial abilities were probably impaired for good and even though he could still speak fluently in five languages, he would always struggle to get a T-shirt over his head.

After almost a year of occupational therapy and practice dressing, one morning Helen heard a plea for help: 'I think I'm in a bit of a pickle with my polo shirt.'

Wanting to encourage independence she replied: 'Just keep trying, love, I'm sure you'll get there.'

'Okay.'

A few minutes passed: 'I'm still in a bit of a pickle.'

And he was.

Udo had managed to squeeze his entire head through the slender sleeve of a polo shirt. It must have been like travelling down the birth canal and we've never fully understood how he achieved it because it took an age to 'un-birth' him.

Helen and the kids had assumed that dressing with an impaired left arm would be a relatively easy task – after all, we'd each had a go and discovered that it was awkward but possible. But we had fully functioning right arms and legs and we had an awareness of our left limbs and we were sensitive to touch. Udo had no awareness of his left limb, no sensitivity to touch and a marked weakness in the left side of his body. Impaired spatial ability and motor skills meant that even Udo's right hand was no longer as agile as it had been and his ability to judge distance and hold shape in mind was not good, so slipping on a sweater or his trousers was no easy task despite having a 'good' right arm and leg. This was why, months after discharge, Udo putting on a T-shirt could still be something of a shocking spectacle: watching him lose awareness of his left hand and arm as it disappeared under the cloth (with no sensory awareness it really was a case of 'out of sight, out of mind'); watching him struggle to distinguish arm hole and neck opening, even though these were very familiar concepts; watching him wrestle with the simple manoeuvre necessary to slip a vest over the head, a manoeuvre he'd been doing for sixty years. And this took up so much concentration that it was not possible to hold a conversation at the same time. How things had changed.

After discharge, there is only limited NHS physiotherapy available to most brain injury victims and after a brief intervention by an outstanding community therapist, we had to recruit private therapists. For us the PIP allowance just covered the cost of weekly sessions but that won't be the case for everyone. We were also fortunate because Udo was in the know – former colleagues had set up a private service and we approached them with absolute confidence and were spared the experience of recruiting people who fell short of the mark. Once set up, the visits were pure joy for Udo – the conversations were characterised by talk of potential, there was a friendly camaraderie between former colleagues, and a still frail Udo felt valued and hopeful that he might regain mobility, stamina and a modicum of independence.

The house now looked different – there was a key-safe at the front door, a stairlift in the hall, additional handrails throughout the house, all manner of grab bars and supports in the bathroom. A challenge for house-proud, aesthetic Udo to tolerate but essential for safety. Even so, there were stumbles and a year on from his stroke, Udo fell, head first, on to a stone floor. One of Udo's nightmares had become a reality – and in A&E at some ungodly hour in the morning we were told that the brain scan probably showed a new brain bleed. We both knew all too well what a brain bleed could lead to.

'That's just how it is. Sorry,' said the brusque medic who then left us to sit with this devastating piece of news. Helen dreaded the worsening of Udo's condition, wondered how long he'd remain conscious, wondered if this time the bleed would kill him. Luckily for Udo he was not completely aware, so he wasn't so worried, he was just tired, and he mumbled and dozed with Helen sitting by his bedside. It might now sound rather melodramatic but Helen, looking at Udo propped up in his hospital bed, couldn't shake off the final scene of one of his favourite films, *Blade Runner*. It's raining and the android Roy Batty slowly powers down, his speech weakens and then he quietly dies. In those early hours Helen wondered if that was how it would be.

In the end, Udo was very lucky, and he didn't suffer another brain haemorrhage, although he did have terrible vertigo for a couple of months. It was so severe that every morning he would sit up in bed only to be thrown back by the vertigo and when he stood he sometimes 'saw' the room flip 90 degrees, so the opposite wall became the floor and the bedside chair seemed to hang off the wall. This frequently made him feel nauseous as well as unsteady. Quite predictably, all this seriously undermined his confidence in standing and walking, but at least we weren't returned to square one (or worse) and there was even a silver lining to the awful experience. Before the night of the fall we'd reached a point of despairing about Udo's progress – we were beginning to spiral into self-pity and envy – but that morning in A&E we discovered how much worse things could have been and we were reminded to cherish what we had. Udo was still with us and he had his speech and we could communicate. We knew that not everyone has that post-stroke. We were also again reminded of the marvellous aspects of the NHS, the constructive and supportive neurology staff, the kindly but so efficient paramedics, the nocturnal nursing staff who were relentlessly cheery on our shift. Mercifully, the rather blunt, and probably very tired, doctor was the exception.

Something else that cheered Helen was that, since discharge, Udo's rehabilitation focus had shifted so that he had more of a balance between physical and cognitive recovery. More and more he was looking for a purpose in life. At last he was concerned about being able to perform mental tasks well again and he began to read more academic papers and develop ideas for research. He had so often seen this pattern of progress in his own patients – the home environment propelled the psychological rehabilitation. Perhaps this is because being at home reminds a person more powerfully of their former self and Udo's former self was a very active doctor and he began to reflect on that part of himself. His first goal of recovery had been to return home, but a close second was to return to meaningful work in some form.

It was on his return home that the meetings with Occupational Health and with a specialist Vocational Rehabilitation service had begun. Both services promised to try their best to find him some form of work, but neither could give a guarantee. That was fair, unsettling but fair. Initially the meetings held hope that Udo would be robust enough to resume relevant part-time work and various options were discussed. But there was a marked dichotomy between the creative approach of the departments of HR, Occupational Health and Vocational Rehabilitation, and the pragmatic view of the medical hierarchy. The latter, quite understandably, had a practical remit – to resume a safe, time- and cost-efficient service as soon as possible. Udo knew that he could not return to his previous job but sensed that he was being eased out of the NHS altogether. This fed the low mood that now pervaded our lives. In his book, *My Year Off*, Robert McCrum describes how his life began again a year after his stroke, how new opportunities arose. This will happen for some, but not all.

Our experience was that one year on opportunities and the light at the end of the tunnel were receding.

Udo still had no proprioception, no true awareness of where his left limbs were. So, he moved his left limbs very, very consciously and very slowly without being able to feel their position, without being aware whether or not his foot had touched the ground. He could still only potter, exhausted after 20 or so metres, clearly struggling to walk. It was made harder because the spasticity in his left leg caused marked shaking (called clonus). Sometimes this was so violent that his whole body shook, and he feared he'd fall again. Yet another irony in his life was that nearly twenty years earlier he had established a Spasticity Clinic in Oxford that administered muscular Botox injections to ease clonus. It was usually very effective, and his patients were almost universally effusive in their gratitude. Now he understood why. Clonus is disabling and relief from it makes a huge difference.

Clonus affected Udo's ability to walk and it made him self-conscious and then he couldn't focus and then he was vulnerable to falling. It was also physically draining and physical exhaustion immediately led to extreme mental fatigue, so his cognitive capability was compromised by his physical weakness. When this happened the wit, wisdom and focus of Udo was lost until he'd rested enough for his body to recharge his mental batteries and overcome the fatigue. Fatigue was still a monster blocking recovery at every stage, relentlessly sabotaging physical, cognitive and emotional recovery.

One year after the stroke, we invited a few friends over to celebrate Udo's survival and recovery. It was not a 'good' day. We were haunted by the memories of the morning of the stroke and one year on it was as if they'd been re-digitalised for the occasion. Udo was tired and withdrawn and we dreaded the arrival of friends because this would almost certainly drain what little energy he had and set him up for the worst and most upsetting of days – the days that our kids called the 'zombie' days. Yet something novel happened. Friends arrived, and Udo brightened up, seemed energised by his visitors, and engaged in conversations. This was a significant change and a positive one. It meant that now he could benefit from social interactions rather than be depleted by them.

Something similar happened a few months later when we had a small birthday party for Udo: he held court, his attention was sustained, his conversation was very coherent, and his mood was lifted.

It was not all joy, one year on, though. The wheelchair, once considered a transitory tool in recovery, was still an absolute necessity if we left the house. The stairlift, initially seen as a temporary device, was also a firm fixture, although Udo tried to make light of his disappointment in needing it. One morning as he slowly descended the particularly steep curve of the stairs, dangling in mid-air, he announced his arrival: 'I look like Zeus making an entry in a second-rate pantomime.'

Udo was still prone to episodes of his mind wandering and not really thinking straight. One afternoon we were walking from the car to a friend's house. Suddenly, without any explanation, he halted mid-stroll.

'Udo, what is it?'

'Just day-dreaming,' he replied, as if this were the most natural thing in the world.

Because of these odd interludes it became all too easy to assume that Udo wasn't quite with it but so often we were wrong, and we were quite rightly put in our place. Our daughter was once gently critical of him for not thinking quickly and a hurt Udo responded: 'I've had a stroke, but I've not lost my marbles, you know.' She agreed that he had not lost his marbles then added: '. . . but they do roll more slowly now, Dad.' Like her father she used humour to keep the disappointments at bay.

By now progress had slowed and it was imperceptible from day to day, week to week. Fortunately, those who visited every few weeks or months noticed shifts for the better and chivvied us on, but we struggled to chivvy ourselves on. Soon after the year anniversary, despondency began to set in, so it was little comfort when a colleague informed us that: 'Years two to five are the worst.'

There was no doubt that re-entering the real world for us had been difficult: the chronicity of Udo's difficulties, the roller-coaster course of progress and most of all the ongoing uncertainty about his recovery and his/our future.

At Christmas, Helen sent out the usual annual greeting, but this time it included a plea for an end to our *Annus horribilis*. We are still not sure what inspired this rather pretentious request, but our PC was having none of it. Its spell-check didn't accommodate Latin and twenty-odd greetings had gone out before Helen spotted what the auto-correct had been up to.

We entered 2018 as a family, which was such an improvement on the year before, but bad memories continued to haunt us. Udo still had flashbacks to some of his most horrendous experiences, in particular the shock of thinking that his arm had been torn from his shoulder. These very vivid memories were so intense that for a moment he felt as though he was back there again, reliving it. One of Udo's flashbacks was of waking with the intense shoulder pain, certain that his left arm was now a detached, dead limb. Flashbacks can suddenly intrude on our thinking and in an instant cause distress. If emotional lability is still an active symptom, there can be tears too. Udo's flashbacks were not what you would call persistent but when they happened, they were intense. Because of our professional backgrounds we understood what they were, yet they were still very upsetting. We could only imagine what it must be like for someone who doesn't know about flashbacks, the terror that they might feel and perhaps even the fear that they are losing their mind.

Flashbacks are just one symptom of a condition known as post-traumatic stress disorder (PTSD); other symptoms are feeling on edge, worrying and avoidance of thoughts or situations that trigger thinking about the trauma. Sometimes PTSD involves emotional numbing (feeling nothing or feeling emotionally blunted). Udo probably didn't have these symptoms severely enough to merit a psychiatric diagnosis of PTSD, but he did have some of the symptoms, particularly flashbacks and being on edge. Udo was much more of a worrier now than he'd ever been, constantly on the lookout for danger, easily startled when he was walking, constantly fearful of falling. This took pleasure out of so many social outings because Udo would be sitting in the wheelchair or taking a short walk to a friend's front door consumed with fears that the wheelchair might career off the pavement and under a car or that he would tumble and get another head injury. He became happier to sit at home and avoid the stress of worrying about falling. This is a typical response to fear, but avoidance only makes things harder, so we had to keep pushing ourselves to visit others, to go to the pub once a week, to face the stress of attending public events. And it always paid off; Udo felt more positive and little by little rebuilt his confidence.

It's possible that some stroke survivors experience PTSD or sub-clinical PTSD and there is a danger that a person might conclude that they are weak or crazy and be too ashamed or scared to ask for help. It's worth noting that post-traumatic symptoms can be delayed, and it is not unusual to get them weeks or months after the traumatic event and this peculiar timing can make them seem even more alarming. Some information about flashbacks can at least put a person's mind at rest and there is quite a lot of material on websites. The most important thing to know about flashbacks is that they are a perfectly usual after-effect of a strong emotional experience. We all have them from time to time and they tend to fade and even if they don't they are relatively easy to manage with the help of a psychological therapist. The key to easing the flashbacks is to try to relax about them. Easier said than done, of course, but the first step in doing this is to remind oneself that they are normal. The next step is to create a dialogue with the flashback, 'updating' it, remembering that this is a bad memory and the reality now is that one survived.

So, when Udo 'felt' and 'saw' the severed arm, he would say to himself: 'This is a memory. My arm is still part of me and it's starting to work again.'

More than a year on and our lives had become differently difficult, the challenges that we faced were no longer those of the early days or the inpatient period but there were new obstacles. Udo had day after day of fatigue and indecisiveness and it was often too easy to yet again let social opportunities slip, have a day off from tedious arm and leg exercises, tolerate lengthy snoozes in the afternoon. We learnt that we couldn't ignore them or put them off; we had to keep applying ourselves to Project Kischka: actively supporting Udo's physical rehabilitation exercises, actively supporting his return to meaningful occupation and – just as important – actively supporting the kids in their readjustment to our situation.

Other things held us back, for example Helen's tendency to assume the worst if things did not go smoothly. Her fears would then be picked up by Udo and this undermined his confidence. One morning Udo had again forgotten something minor like bringing his sweater downstairs or leaving his walking stick in the usual place and Helen was panicking because surely this degree of forgetfulness so long after the stroke meant that he'd never recover. To make the morning even more stressful she couldn't find the car keys. This was because she had left them in the ignition overnight – in a car that stands in the open street. However, 'That's just old age, Udo, we all get forgetful ...' Nothing to worry about. Two standards: a realistic one for Helen and a tougher one for Udo. On another occasion she inadvertently knocked Udo's confidence by observing (and worrying) that it was taking him an alarmingly long time to learn the routine for using the stairlift. Udo agreed that some time had passed and yet he could not reliably carry out this routine. In part he attributed this to the difficulty he now expected when faced with learning a spatial routine, but he also pointed out that he was handicapped in his learning because on nine out of ten occasions, Helen had again forgotten to switch on the stairlift downstairs thus leaving him stranded at the top of the house trying to call her from his mobile phone. The truth was that Helen's memory was stress impaired and she accepted that, but when Udo had memory problems she panicked.

Helen's catastrophic view of life not only risked undermining Udo's confidence but if she wasn't careful it impacted on the kids, who would pick up either on Mum's worry or on Dad's distress or both. We learnt to identify this chain of upset as 'domestic dominoes' and Helen tried to catch it early. The fears that we have as a stroke sufferer or a carer can so easily drive panic and misinterpretation and we need to be able to recognise it, to stand back and get things in perspective. Of course, it's not a very comfortable position if the conclusion is that one's memory is much worse than the person who has had the stroke.

Actually, by now Helen had a full house of post-stroke symptoms – fatigue, confusion, forgetfulness and an emotional lability equal to Udo's. She was officially ditzy, evidenced by events such as the supermarket walk of shame returning goods to shelves because she'd forgotten her purse or offering teetotal Udo a lively cocktail one morning because what she thought was a generous dash of elderflower cordial was a glug of white wine. There is often no real respite for the carers and it takes its toll. Thank goodness for a sympathetic boss and a job that granted a good deal of autonomy and the prospect of working from home because this eased the stress.

Nonetheless, a new experience proved a real challenge for Helen: envy. She had often wished for things that others enjoyed – long legs, social confidence, the getaway in Tuscany – but these were all things she'd never had, and it was easy to accept that they weren't to be. Now she envied those who had what we had lost: a capable dad, financial security, the option of holding hands and walking over Magdalen Bridge. Envy was toxic and draining, almost as draining as living with uncertainty. In the end it helped to deal with it like managing uncertainty and worry – if there's nothing you can do about it, mentally park it and walk away. (In Chapter 7 you can read more about dealing with worry.)

And the children? Since adjusting to their father's return home, the teens seemed more settled, there was more laughter, but it was fragile, and it still wasn't easy. Our girl no longer referred to the 'living bereavement' of the early months but Dad still wasn't quite Dad and she clearly mourned the loss. Her brother still didn't speak about his father at school and asked Helen not to say anything to teachers on parents' evening. We noticed that he no longer invited friends over but relied more and more on communicating with them via his PlayStation. Perhaps this is normal teen behaviour, but perhaps it's a young man in denial. We would never know because he didn't talk about his feelings. He did scavenge a lot of midnight ice cream, though.

Friends and professionals began asking Udo if he was depressed because his mood was so flat. He wasn't depressed, but he was grieving. The hope that keeps grief at bay was losing that battle. As the rate of recovery slowed, so doors closed. Walking to the end of the road – not looking so likely now; driving again – not going to happen so we'd sold his car; returning to work – the prospect kept receding until, just after Christmas 2017, Udo decided that he would have to resign from his job. The fatigue was not easing, and it affected his sustained attention and mental alacrity, so he could not possibly return to his former clinical post. In effect, this meant bidding farewell to a hard-earned career as a very active medical doctor long before he wanted to, and this was a crushing blow. Retiring was the hardest decision he had ever made, and he reflected on all those times as a doctor he'd encouraged a patient to take early retirement, not fully appreciating the devastating meaning that it could have. With hindsight he would have spent more time discovering what giving up the hope of returning to work really meant to his patients.

In the Kischka family there had been a family tradition of training as a doctor. Initially Udo had thought that he would become a psychiatrist. He wanted to understand the workings of the human mind as well as the body and so he first studied psychology for five years in Germany. He then applied to medical schools. He was offered a place in Amsterdam and promptly set about learning Dutch to take up the training there. Clearly, he'd invested in his career and if truth be told he never wanted to stop practising as a medical doctor – he loved the work and he'd worked hard to get there. The realisation that this was to end hit him hard, his mood dipped and with it the volume of his voice, the strength in his left side and his motivation to maintain his rehabilitation. He grew despondent and hopeless. He lost his appetite and became pale and thin. He couldn't see a meaningful future beyond the family.

It took a casual comment from a Danish neurologist friend to kick-start hope: 'What you have going for you, Udo, is plasticity and tenacity.' This was and is true: his brain was capable of more development; there was still work to be done, progress to be had.

6

Reclaiming Life After a Stroke: 'He Did Plateau at Ninety'

Eighteen months passed.

As the recovery rate slows and each day looks like the day before and the week before and even the month before, it is easy to assume that there will be no more progress. Helen was in this frame of mind when she started talking with a local shopkeeper. 'Oh, my uncle had a terrible stroke when he was seventy, a really bad one,' the shopkeeper revealed. 'We thought that was that but, you know, he never stopped improving. Every time we visited there would be some change, some progress.' This was a well-timed and heartening comment and then she added: 'Tell a lie – he did plateau at ninety.'

Nonetheless, thanks to brain plasticity, we still have over twenty-five years of Udo's progress to look forward to. Given his father was working until he was ninety (and then continued to live a full if more sedentary life) it was reasonable to assume that Udo might live long and that it was crucial to find a life with meaning and purpose. Losing the professional identity that it had taken him an adulthood to forge shattered him and being so physically reduced meant that options for purposeful activity were now limited.

Weekly physical rehabilitation sessions reminded us that Udo could achieve more independence, even if he would never run up and down the stairs again, and visiting friends observed that he was growing more alert at each visit. Family members and friends were so pleased for Udo, but he remained subdued. We wondered why. He recalled times when, as a doctor, he had given feedback on progress to his patients and he was surprised that they were not more pleased to learn of their achievements. Now he understood: he hardly ever compared his progress to what he was doing a month ago but instead he considered his abilities before his stroke. This is still the case and far too frequently the satisfaction of progress is diminished by the memory of what was and what has been lost.

Despite this outlook, it seemed reasonable to hope that he could achieve more. Our forays to museums and exhibitions had been curtailed by the cold weather that literally pained Udo, but now spring was here the air was merely damp not frosty, and we could resume cultural pursuits. Armed with recently acquired membership cards we could even jump the queue at the local museum and the independent cinema, both of which were more than wheelchair friendly. It really was worth fighting the monsters of apathy and fatigue because the visits always paid off. They reconnected us to a world beyond the comfortable chair in the corner of our conservatory and often forced Udo to stretch himself intellectually and physically – and without that he was not going to make the most of brain plasticity.

Finding a hobby helped. It was a new avenue to explore and Udo chose to research a seventeenth-century princess – Liselotte of Heidelberg. Udo had grown up hearing stories of this remarkable royal from his father who was a historian. She was much loved in her city of origin and although she seems to have evoked little interest outside her hometown, Udo had become just as enchanted as his father before him.

At nineteen years of age, Princess Liselotte of the Palatinate was married to the brother of Louis XIV, the Sun King, in the hope that this alliance would protect her father's lands. Sadly, the plan did not work and in 1688 Louis XIV ordered his armies to make the Palatinate 'a desert' and later Liselotte's beloved Heidelberg itself was razed to the ground. She was devastated by the loss of her home and loved ones, and she felt deeply betrayed by the French royal family. We know this because she was an avid letter writer. Her letters give a fascinating and often entertaining insight into life at court, but they also record her hardships: the death of her young son, the loss of her father, the infidelities of her husband and the terrible loneliness and isolation that she suffered at Versailles. Yet Liselotte remained determined to survive, to speak her mind and to maintain her moral standards.

The Liselotte project not only offered Udo an opportunity to read and write in his first language and to improve his use of the laptop and develop his mental multitasking skills, her story of coping in adversity was inspiring and, corny as it might sound, if we can find inspiration we tend to look forwards rather than dwelling on the present. The project also gave him a chance to work with his father, which further helped him feel grounded and connected to the world.

Research stretching back to the 1970s shows us that when we feel adrift and vulnerable the sense of being connected and having a 'safe base' can be the difference between coping and not coping. As we noted earlier in the book, just having a single, trustworthy person in whom to confide has been shown to be enough to protect us against the fears and miseries that can hold us back. Udo was fortunate in having his Oxford family and active links with his Heidelberg family, all of which strengthened his confidence and his resolve to make progress. Some people won't be so lucky and may need to work harder to find the social connections that will give them a sense of being grounded and supported. There are many organisations that set up support for survivors of stroke and other brain injuries (there is a list of these in Chapter 9) and it can be worth striving to join them. For some this will mean overcoming shyness, fears or hopelessness; for others it will be a more physical challenge of overcoming immobility or the obstacle of fatigue.

The organisation that we had most contact with was the Oxfordshire branch of Headway, but there are many other organisations and charities nationwide. They typically provide daily, affordable, programmes that give attendees a chance to continue with their rehabilitation amongst a group of people with whom they can identify. Staff frequently help with form filling and transport, two huge obstructions. Long before his stroke, Udo had been a supporter of Headway Oxfordshire in a professional capacity. He had been an advisor and trustee, he helped organise training for the staff and had worked hard in order to improve the interface between the hospital services and the charity. Now it offered him a chance to be reinstated as an expert in his field, even more expert since he'd had his own brain bleed. Udo could, at least in part, revive his role as a stroke specialist. It couldn't have come at a better time.

He was invited to give presentations to small groups of Headway users and professionals. He first practised with the vocational rehabilitation team and when he'd gathered enough confidence he put on his grey suit for the first time in nearly a year and a half and returned to the stage as Professor Kischka. He discovered that he could comfortably perform for an hour and accommodate a few questions. These brief teaching stints were very well received and helped to rebuild a flagging optimism and self-confidence. They were a powerful reminder that he still had a role to play in his chosen professional field. His useful life was not over and there were still things that could give his life meaning beyond being part of a family.

One of his presentations for colleagues was inspired by his early experiences in hospital. Recalling what he had concluded in those early days, he called it: *Stroke: I knew @*&% all!* It gave a vivid account of how his professional expectations had differed from his personal reality as a stroke survivor literally from the first day of his admission. This one proved to be so relevant that he was asked to present it again . . . and again.

He was also invited to write short papers about his experiences as a doctor transformed into a patient. A friend suggested the title: *From Medical Consultant to Bed-blocker.* Then there were the research ideas. Prior to the stroke Udo had been a keen collaborator in rehabilitation research but with time on his hands and his own experience he now had many more ideas about aspects of rehabilitation that could be more closely studied. In particular, he was more interested in the relevance of active rehabilitation months and even years after stroke. It was around this time that one of his former research colleagues invited him to rejoin the University of Oxford stroke research team and Udo couldn't have been more keen. The chance of putting his research ideas into action might now become a reality. Later still, a lively group of researchers at Oxford Brookes University not only invited him to join them as an Affiliate Fellow but offered him some desk space. Perhaps doors were beginning to open.

It is said that the second year is particularly hard – by now most of the very obvious recovery has been made and we learn what we are likely to have to live with. For some, the second year will be a satisfying almost-return to old times, perhaps with more appreciation and respect for life, but for us there remained a sense of disappointment. We were still far too often waking up dissatisfied, going through the day frustrated and returning to bed looking forward to a few hours of oblivion – if we were lucky. We were still shocked that progress could be so easily thwarted. Within a short time, progress that had taken weeks to amass could seemingly disappear because Udo had been forced to reduce his intensive exercising because of stress, fatigue or illness. We came to realise that Udo's fourteen-minute walk to and from the end of our crescent was the equivalent of an athlete's four-minute mile. It actually stretched him beyond his natural capabilities, and he could not keep it up without Olympian dedication. Eventually he had to make a decision either to dedicate his waking hours to doing a lot of exercise to keep up that fourteen-minute walk or to take it easier and settle for less.

We felt guilty for not being more chipper, but all four of us were still adjusting and we were exhausted; there had been no time off for emotional recovery since the stroke and that takes its toll. Udo recalled a very apt German saying: '*Die Läenge trägt die Last.*' 'The duration carries the burden.'

We don't want to give the impression that it was endlessly grim because there were hopeful times and laughter, too, but we want to give an honest picture of our lives months and months after the stroke when signs of recovery are subtle, emotional exhaustion has become the norm and circumstances change.

At school some of the teachers were wondering why the kids were not performing better: after all, '. . . your dad's home now. He survived, and the stroke was a long time ago.' The reality is that each day is a reminder of loss and each day is still laced with fears. Many of the questions that we had eighteen months ago still came to mind: How are we going to carry on like this? Will Udo ever be himself again? But now we felt uncomfortable expressing them; we felt that we should be coping better – and to the outside world it looked as though we were managing. We lost count of the times we were told that we were 'marvellous' for coping and 'doing really well'. This was not so evident behind closed doors where tempers were easily frayed, thoughts could be dark, anger could simmer and from time to time there were tears:

'I want to be whole again, Helen.'

'Mum, it scares me when Dad is a Muppet.'

'I feel as if I am no longer a person.'

'I hate this. I can't bear this way of being . . .'

'Not again . . .'

In an attempt to manage the household efficiently Helen fell into the trap of becoming far too bossy and Udo felt humiliated, diminished, and there were angry outbursts that could harm our chances of regaining a family life, so we tried very hard to understand why we were getting on each other's nerves and we certainly apologised a lot. Luckily Udo is an understanding and forgiving man and, although Helen would mutter for some while after a row, she learnt to let go of grudges so that we could move on.

There were good reasons why our relationship was now more strained. The simple fact that we were dealing with the stress of change, and for Udo this often felt unbearable, was sufficient to explain a good deal of tension, but there were other explanations and it helped to become aware of these, too.

You might remember that in Chapter 3 we said that character traits can get exaggerated after a stroke, so if your loved one did something that irritated you before the stroke and now it is exaggerated . . . Well, you can imagine what it's like for a stressed family. In the past, when something was 'lost' in our house, Helen had asked: 'Have you looked or have you "Kischka-looked"?' Father, daughter and son typically (and passionately) claimed that they'd searched and whatever it was wasn't there. Yet when Mum looked behind, beneath or beyond objects she usually found what was missing. It drove her mad – for nearly two decades it had driven her mad. After the stroke Udo's 'Kischka-looking' was exaggerated. Helen should have responded to the cry: 'It's not here!' with compassion, appreciating that in addition to all the other challenges he had, Udo's ability to search for things was now very compromised by his attention problems and the hemineglect. Instead, the cry triggered an almost knee-jerk reaction of judgemental eye-rolling and sighing. As you might predict, this hurt and eventually angered Udo. It took effort to break free of this well-honed habit and it's still a work in progress because at times of stress the twenty-year-old response kicks back in. That's the nature of learning and over-rehearsal – practice, practice, practice builds an automatic response. It is a principle behind rehabilitation, but in this case, it was working against us.

Aaron T. Beck, the father of CBT, wrote that behind unwarranted anger in relationships lay fear or hurt and this made sense to us, too. For example, Helen might notice that Udo hadn't done something or other and the fear would kick in –'He's not making progress; life is never going to improve for us . . .' – and her cross reaction would hurt Udo, who didn't deserve to be reprimanded and sometimes he would bark back. Then Helen would feel righteously angry and off we'd go. We tried not to fall into this trap in the first place but when we did we introduced a cooling- off period asap. We were helped by a daughter who, quite rightly, took us to task when the bickering began. She was now an older teenager able to express her disappointment in her parents, but some kids like her brother will suffer in silence, perhaps feeling very vulnerable.

It's yet another sad fact that many relationships don't survive the stress of adjusting following a brain injury, but fortunately Udo had continued to work with a clinical psychologist from the vocational rehabilitation services who was also a talented couples therapist. A few joint sessions with him gave us invaluable guidance and perspective and an abiding message was: 'Put effort into a new game plan because things are different now. *Make a new life happen.*' So that's what we've been trying to do since: work together to make a new life happen. It is not the life we want, or ever wanted, and it's not an easy life, but we reminded ourselves that it could be worse, and it could be better. We listed the 'at least's yet again and made plans to stop us stagnating and to unite us in this shared project. We timetabled shared activities and tried at least to hold hands more often, even when the day was busy and we were both tired. But even now it can require conscious thought and it has really needed both of us to commit to it. What made it easier was still being able to value each other: from day one Helen marvelled at Udo's dignity and fortitude in the face of his hated condition and he was deeply moved by the caring he received from his wife and family. But we needed to remember to tell each other this.

As time went by we continued to see more progress, and this inevitably helped our relationship. By nineteen months, Udo's walking was becoming more elegant, even if stamina remained a problem. He began to get a very vague sensation in his left leg and foot when he moved – to be honest it was very, very vague but it was an awareness that didn't used to be there and a clear reminder that his brain had not given up on the repair work. Around the same time, we noticed an improvement in his bare-foot walking. Usually he wore a heavy ankle splint, nicknamed

'Robocop' because it looked like part of that character's armoured costume. Udo hated it because, although it held his ankle firm, easing the clonus and ensuring that he didn't wobble, it was heavy, uncomfortable and restricted development in his foot and ankle movements. So, from time to time, he would go barefoot across the bedroom with Helen watching closely, fearful of another fall. At first his big toe had dropped and dragged and seemed to claw the floor as he walked, now there was little or no drop and the walking movement looked more natural. Again, we have brain plasticity to thank but also ongoing rehab exercises guided by our weekly therapists.

For months Udo had been sitting on the edge of the bed, following physiotherapy orders, dutifully raising and lowering his left toes before he turned in for the night. It was a safe exercise, so Helen didn't feel the need to watch and besides, it seemed to make very little difference so there was no thrill of progress and for weeks she neither encouraged this nor bothered to pay much attention. She was impressed by Udo's dedication to an exercise that seemed too slight to make any difference but thank goodness he had the good sense to keep at it. As a rehab specialist himself he knew that there are no quick fixes, especially by the second year, so perseverance is crucial; he also knew that 'slight' does not mean 'ineffective' because good physical rehab is often about precision and the development of the correct, small movement. His commitment and belief were now paying off because he was regaining fluid movement from his ankle right through to his toes, a smooth movement that was essential for 'proper' walking. His hemi-neglect and hemiparesis meant that he could only do this if he could actually see his foot, but it was such an achievement we were not going to be critical.

Udo was also walking more with a slim walking stick – not far, as he still ran out of stamina quite quickly. His weekly outdoor stroll (40 metres) was taking slightly less time and he was pottering about the house. So, it would be easy to assume that this movement was increasingly effortless for him; he had always assumed this when he'd seen his own patients practise walking. But once again he knew @*&% all. He had been what we call 'ambulatory' for well over a year but even now it was far from effortless, his experience was of 'wobbling along' never 'walking', so no wonder he remained insecure.

There was an indisputable improvement in the quality of his walking, particularly on a 'good day' when he was not fatigued, ill or stressed. So, it was true that he was gaining skill and confidence but much less quickly than he'd anticipated and with much more fragility. He discovered that walking continued to be effortful and to this day he experiences unease and a fear of falling and he is still exhausted after only a short walk. This is because walking involves an enormous amount of mental and physical coordination, particularly for a person who has a brain lesion where Udo had his. Walking requires a person not to get distracted by sounds or sights, and Udo became more distractible after his stroke. The movement forward has to be incorporated with sensory feedback in order to keep balance and gauge the next step – but Udo still had little or no awareness of the left side of his body, so he had to manage without that feedback. Uneven surfaces pose a terrifying challenge for someone who has lost not only sensory feedback but also depth perception and an awareness of all things to his left. All the elements of movement (strength, balance, alternating limbs), have to be coordinated with planning the walk, problem solving obstacles and dealing with surprises such as a teenage son suddenly practising kickboxing moves: a challenge that exhausted him even this far into rehabilitation. No wonder that Udo couldn't hold a conversation when he was in motion. In fact, we had to ask people not to chat with him lest they disrupted his concentration and caused him to stumble.

If we visited a new place Udo would find himself set back by the challenge of negotiating an unfamiliar surface and the need to make decisions about what direction to take. This happened when we dropped by to see friends and sometimes Udo would stand paralysed on a flat surface that should have been relatively easy for this veteran potterer-about. But faced with insecurity and decision-making he could simply freeze.

Nonetheless, he persevered, determined to become more independent. Mobility was only one sign of increasing independence. By now Udo was also able to dress and disrobe and Helen no longer needed to be a 'dressing coach'. He felt uplifted every time she left him to get on with it: 'Okay, Udo, get yourself dressed and I'll see you downstairs for breakfast.' Left alone, however, he was soon very aware of his physical slowness, and dressing was still a very laborious procedure that did not always go smoothly. This crushed the sense of achievement that he might otherwise have taken from his gradually increasing independence or from an ongoing 'pep' talk from his wife. Alone, he tended to reflect on his limitations, and we realised that although it was good for him to be left to get on with tasks, Udo still very much needed verbal encouragement from the family to drive him on.

He also still needed Helen as a clock-watcher, prompting him to keep going and reminding him of the time. This was not surprising at all. Damage to the basal ganglia and the connections to the frontal areas of the brain (the site of most damage after Udo's stroke) affects our awareness of time passing, especially if the damage is in the right hemisphere. Udo's appreciation of the passing of time was not really improving and without reminders he could slow and stop and not realise that the clock was ticking. This was not always a big problem but on days with deadlines it was a source of stress and friction, and on less structured days it was the reason that Udo lost precious hours. For those trying to reclaim a life worth living this can be a significant obstacle.

Many, many years ago, when Helen was doing her research degree in Oxford, she found part-time work as a psychology assistant at Rivermead Rehabilitation Centre. This was the forerunner of the O.C.E. and it was a collection of old buildings sited by the River Thames. It was where Udo came to work in the late 1990s and where he is remembered for saving a patient who had jumped into the river, remembered less because of his courage and more because he was wearing an expensive suit at the time. When Helen worked there, her boss was an ingenious clinical psychologist (now deservedly a professor) who had a talent for resolving practical problems simply and efficiently. Therefore, back in those days before smartphones and smartwatches, she encouraged patients with memory problems to hang notebooks round their necks so that they could immediately write down the things that they might otherwise forget; she championed clunky digital watches that rang alarms as reminders; she advocated lists of to-dos pinned to the wall. All very practical and affordable and doable. So, when Helen was faced with problems such as Udo's lack of awareness of time she tried to channel her former boss.

As a result, we began using reminders on Udo's smartphone (such as setting alarms to wake him and prompt him at ten-minute intervals that time was passing) and alarms to remind him to take regular exercise during the day. Typically, Udo got used to the sound of the alarms and they quickly lost their potency. Therefore, our teen girl made it her business to discover the phone's most annoying and unpleasant sounds so that Dad would be highly motivated to pay attention and switch off the offensive noise. We also used Post-its on the laptop that had reminders of the day's to-dos and we ensured that his watch was on his right wrist so that there was less chance that it would be neglected. This helped, but only somewhat because we were up against the challenge of the site and extent of Udo's brain lesion – there was a limit to how much awareness he could regain. We still use many reminders, but time-keeping remains a source of difficulty and occasional tensions in the household. The enduring fatigue and apathy haven't helped either.

Although the fatigue was improving, and Udo could now sustain his attention throughout meetings with academic colleagues and with friends, as soon as the event was over he was exhausted, spent. Even now the physical and psychological demands of talking required a great deal of effort and it would wear him out. Just before the two-year anniversary of the stroke we had guests from the US and a long and very enjoyable evening of reminiscing where Udo was on top form, fully engaged and genuinely enjoying himself for over six hours. The next day he slept until mid-afternoon and barely held a conversation with his family for the rest of that day – or the next. Such was his fatigue and his need for time to recharge his batteries. We got used to this pattern of Udo being lively and engaged – his old self – until our guests left. Having seen them to the door, Helen would return to an Udo burnt out from the strain of it all. She and the kids often felt short-changed because Dad seemed to put more effort into being alert for others and we had to remind ourselves that no one could keep up the gargantuan effort it took Udo to maintain prolonged conversation and that it was good that he felt that his home and family provided a safe enough base for him to relax into exhaustion when necessary.

It was unclear if the apathy was getting better, though, and this was still a very frustrating consequence of the stroke for the entire family. There is an old joke:

Question: What's the difference between ignorance and apathy?
Answer: Don't know. Don't care.

This is such a wrong representation of apathy. It's not about not caring. In Udo's case, the parts of the brain that switch on initiation were not working well and although he might genuinely want to do something, might genuinely care about something, he simply couldn't get going. It was very apparent when Udo had been home for a few weeks and he was able to sit up in bed, swing his feet to the floor and – in principle – stand up. But he didn't stand. He sat, and he sat. Eventually he would say: 'Helen, tell me to stand. Say, "Ready, steady, stand-up."' And with this familiar instruction from the O.C.E. he was immediately able to overcome the initiation block and rise to standing. The external prompt is less necessary now, but Udo still often coaches himself to start activities like getting out of the chair and we sometimes hear him quietly repeating the words of his physiotherapist from the hospital: 'Nose over toes and up he goes.'

Apathy has been horribly frustrating for him, especially as he felt that it was out of character and out of his control. A person with apathy can quite wrongly feel lazy and they can be disappointed because they can't fulfil their desires and it's very testing for those around who don't understand why this person just isn't getting on with it – doesn't he care? It doesn't make sense to the observer: it didn't make sense to us. Udo would say that he wanted to work on upper limb exercises or on editing a paper, and an hour later he hadn't begun. It was hard for us to appreciate that it wasn't that he couldn't be bothered; he simply couldn't get going and if we were to help him, then energy was best placed in prompting and encouraging rather than nagging an already disappointed man.

By now we did seem to have fewer setbacks, fewer periods of 'losing' Udo but when they happened they could be just as dramatic as they had been over a year ago. The heatwave of 2018 heralded a sharp decline in Udo's behaviour, movement and cognitive functioning. He grew increasingly fatigued, his voice was a whisper, his head almost perpetually twisted to the right, the daily practice walk took longer, multitasking grew more difficult, his mood was dipping, he was living in the past again, his appetite diminished, he was more forgetful, and Helen found herself once again using a phrase she'd used when he was in the O.C.E.: 'Think it through, Udo.' He did less and less and again seemed to be receding from the family. He was tired, exhausted and aware that he was unravelling again. This alarmed him, then annoyed him, then it drained him, and he gave up the fight to stay awake. He closed his eyes and drifted into semi-sleep, because this was yet another reminder of how things were so much worse than they had been before the stroke and it robbed him of hope that he could regain a life resembling his former existence.

As part of him reclaiming his life, we had set up a visit to Heidelberg. Udo's kind relatives would accompany him there and the rest of us would join him a couple of weeks later. He was now so muddled and exhausted that Helen began to wonder if it would be possible for him to go but we went ahead. Helen dropped him off at the airport and we braced ourselves for news of a terrible journey and Udo feeling dreadful. The call from Germany came through to Oxford in the early evening of the day he arrived in Heidelberg and Udo was a man transformed. He'd discovered that he could travel, that he could board a plane and his homeland – and therefore his German family – was still within reach. His voice was already stronger, his thinking clearer and his mood certainly improved. Whilst there he went to the theatre a couple of times and attended a wedding ceremony and lengthy party and by the time Helen and the kids joined him his appetite had increased enough for his trousers to be noticeably better fitting. The experience of taking a vacation, catching up with old friends, eating in the family's restaurant, whilst also taking rest periods with his father, had worked magic. He felt satisfaction and pride.

So, what did we learn from this?

Not to fall into the trap of inactivity.

Yes, Udo had become more tired and weak in the hot weather but by taking the line of non-stop resting and cutting back on activity we had robbed him of pleasurable activity and any sense of achievement, which in turn demoralised him and brought him down. Heidelberg had restored his well-being instantly. With hindsight we should have kept up moderate activities and made sure that we were doing enough to remind us all that Udo was still making progress. Helen and Udo both tended to pull back from activity when he was tired and too much of this had actually set him back. This was in contrast to a year earlier when Udo overdid things in rehab, and this had similarly exhausting results. So, it is crucial not to overdo things either. If we were going to forge a reasonable existence, if Udo was going achieve his potential, we had to balance helpful activity and rest periods.

It was now a year since Udo's discharge and it seemed a good time to take stock. Although change was slow and subtle, we looked back and could see that it was there. You might recall our disappointment when Udo wasn't up to attending a piano concert soon after he left hospital; well, a year on we booked tickets for the same performer and the circumstances were so different. Not only did Udo now have the mental and physical stamina needed to get to the theatre and listen to the music, he was excited about it, he was looking forward to it and he reflected on the concert afterwards – in short, he was so much more engaged with his world and this felt wonderful to him. He was happy that he and his wife could still share enjoyable experiences and he had a sense of achievement.

Helen, who like the Ancient Mariner had needed to tell her tale as a sort of catharsis, now found the urge was less intense. The daily log had become a weekly log and sometimes forgotten altogether as it became unnecessary to capture the strange goings-on in the family because it all felt less strange and we were now doing more normal things. We were getting used to our new life and Udo was overcoming more obstacles.

As his rehabilitation moved forward we dared to anticipate the time when he would be able to abandon the stairlift or the time when the OT would suggest immobilising his right arm because she had confidence in his ability to use the left one. This is a well-established treatment to overcome non-use of the not-so-good limb. It is understandable that when it is effortful and frustrating to try to carry out a task with a weak hand and arm a person simply uses the 'good' arm. The problem is that the hand and arm that are used get better and better at managing the task, making it less and less likely that the other side is used. This then means that the brain doesn't develop the new pathways necessary for improving functioning of the weak limb – a waste of brain potential. A solution to this is putting the 'good' arm in a sling and the 'good' hand in a mitten so that they become just as frustrating and difficult to use. Thus, the weak arm and hand have to be put to use, and the brain circuitry and physical strength start to develop.

Although Udo would eventually engage in immobilisation exercises, right now it was too soon – his left arm was not yet strong enough or biddable enough to do many daily tasks and it was certainly not going to support him if he fell. But we felt that we were working towards this goal as his formerly 'useless' left arm and hand could now be raised to touch his shoulder, be manoeuvred to unlock the brake on his wheelchair and he'd made us laugh when, without thinking about it, he'd raised his left hand as he demonstrated to a friend: '. . . and I can't move this any more'.

He was getting there but he had realistic expectations about the time it might take. This realistic appraisal was so different from even a year before, and certainly very different from his outlook soon after the stroke when his expectations were often shockingly optimistic. Over-optimism is not unusual following brain injury, particularly when the damage is to the right hemisphere, and in some ways, it was helpful in that it spurred Udo on to make the most of his rehabilitation opportunities. However, as a family we were happier to see him get a realistic grasp of the situation. Yet another sign that he was returning to his old self.

There was also now less uncertainty about the future, so the atmosphere at home was normalising yet we couldn't rid ourselves of the odour of loss and frustration and we wondered if we'd ever feel 'right' again. A friend helped by sharing his own experience of dealing with an unexpected event that left his young family changed for ever. After five years he and his wife looked back and realised they'd come through. In retrospect they didn't know quite how they had dealt with their stress and fear and disappointment, but they realised they had reached a point of true acceptance and the phrase 'This is just how it is' was no longer a platitude used for comfort but words that described how it really was for them and they could live with that. Gone was the anger and envy and they were free to enjoy what they had.

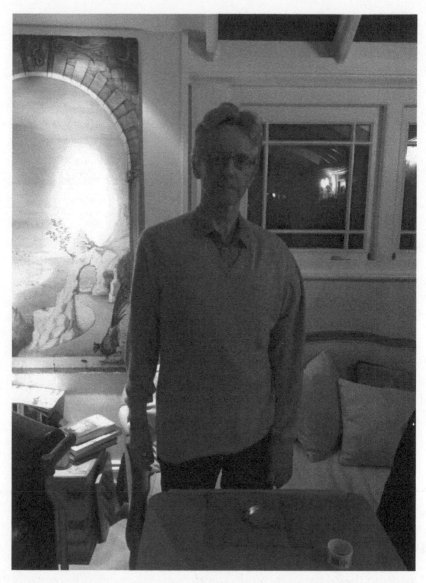

A rehab session at home nearly two years after the stroke

Some will simply gradually reach this state; some will search out self-help resources to get them there, while others will need the help of professionals. We were lucky enough to have had extraordinary professional support in the first year and our ongoing contact with the Vocational Rehabilitation services and

Headway Oxfordshire supported us and enabled us to hope for more as time went on. We were also helped by our knowledge of psychological therapies, CBT in particular of course. In the next chapter Helen describes how we used CBT to help us get on top of some of our difficulties post-stroke. This part of the book might be a helpful taster for those of you who are ready to think about using CBT on your journey of recovery. It is just a brief overview and it might provide sufficient direction for some readers; for others it could be the introduction that leads on to seeking more formal help. Some of you might simply take from it the odd 'top tip' while there might be others who read it and realise that CBT is not for them.

Perhaps the best thing to do is to read through the chapter and see if it appeals to you, without putting yourself under pressure.

7

CBT: Strategies for Survival
Helen Kennerley

Google CBT (cognitive behavioural therapy) and you'll discover that it's a talking therapy that can help you manage your problems by changing the way you think and behave. It was pioneered by Dr Aaron T. Beck in Philadelphia in the 1970s as a treatment for depression, but it rapidly developed into a successful intervention for a wide range of psychological problems: anxieties, anger problems, trauma, relationship difficulties and more.

Stroke patients and their family members will be familiar with the wide range of emotional and psychological challenges that can follow stroke; we certainly were. Like others in our position, we struggled with despair, fear, anger, grief and hopelessness. These are normal responses and CBT wouldn't aim to change realistic distress, but what it can do is help us keep fears, misery and anger in proportion and it can provide a set of strategies for dealing with the emotional difficulties that follow a stroke. That's why we've included this chapter on CBT in the book.

You can try out the techniques now or you can use this chapter later because this might not be the right time for you to be thinking about CBT. In the very early days of Udo's stroke, I was overwhelmed and in shock and I couldn't use many of the strategies outlined here. At that time, I just wanted reassuring information about stroke, distraction and emotional support. I could only start using the techniques of CBT when I'd begun to adjust to our new situation. Then the techniques did help, which is not surprising given that CBT has a background of research showing that it is effective for many people.

CBT is all about supporting and coaching, helping people learn new ways of coping and ultimately becoming experts in managing their own problems. It's a very active form of psychological therapy often involving collecting 'data' in the form of diaries, note-keeping and carrying out surveys. It also encourages trying out new ways of coping to see if new ideas actually work: taking on challenging tasks such as leaving the house, joining a group, being assertive, resisting the urge to check just once more. As a clinical psychologist in training, CBT was the obvious choice for me: I could channel my inner counsellor, researcher and *Blue Peter* presenter.

CBT has stood the test of time. In its fifth decade, it remains an internationally popular and expanding therapy, helped by its having a very respectable research foundation.

All very impressive, but what does CBT entail?

First, CBT helps us recognise our emotional traps, for example:

- the fear that restricts us and further saps confidence;
- the depression behind the withdrawal that then fuels more misery;
- the anger that sabotages plans and creates more frustration;
- the social worry that undermines performance and causes greater anxiety.

These are common traps and there are many more – by now you might be very familiar with some.

Our family's experience was of high levels of anxiety about the future, often coming as a series of questions:

- Will he pull through? Will he have that second stroke? Will the pneumonia kill him?
- Will I always be this disabled?
- How will we afford the care we need?

- Will he ever be his old self again or will we be living with a stranger?
- Will the kids be able to cope – what about their needs?

There were also the depressing and angry questions:

- Why us?
- Why me?
- Why didn't I take more care of myself?
- Was it my fault?

Asking ourselves questions is normal. You will no doubt have your own list of worries and thoughts that knot your stomach and keep you awake at night. CBT can help to take the edge off the intensity of this but only when we have turned questions into statements, only when we have named the fear or distress. So, this is always a first step in CBT, and in itself it can be difficult.

Stating 'I am afraid that he will die' or '. . . that he will always be this disabled' or '. . . we have lost the person we knew and loved' is probably harder than saying, 'What if . . .?' However, it is difficult to either (i) check things out or (ii) use the strategies of CBT unless we have named the thought (or mental image) that drives the distress. This is something to bear in mind as you deal with your own reactions to being a stroke survivor or a loved one or a carer.

When Udo was in intensive care, our son, understandably, concluded that his father could die any day. Unbeknown to us, this stayed with him and haunted him. Only by chance did he articulate it many, many months later. And only at that point was I was able to reassure him that the dangerous days were long since over and he revised his expectations. It was a simple intervention but its impact was striking – he re-engaged with the family, particularly with his father, and his mood and demeanour improved. If only we'd been aware of his fearful thoughts earlier: hindsight will always be a wonderful thing.

Once the statement behind the fear or the misery or the anger is clear, but the problem persists, CBT helps us recognise the thinking and behaviours that create traps.

The way we think (whether this is in words or just mental pictures) colours the way we feel and the way we feel influences the way we think. If an alarming thought such as: 'I will always be this disabled' crosses a man's mind, then he will probably feel scared and his fearfulness will make him even more vulnerable to frightening thoughts.

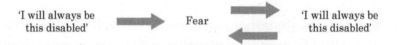

'I will always be this disabled' → Fear → 'I will always be this disabled'

He might now get stuck in the trap of his worries driving fear and fear making him more prone to worries. It's the same when we have miserable thoughts. I found myself getting caught in this trap of hopeless thinking and feelings of misery, especially in the early hours of the morning.

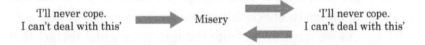

'I'll never cope. I can't deal with this' → Misery → 'I'll never cope. I can't deal with this'

Fears and misery are painful emotions so we all do our best to devise strategies for coping: 'If I ignore it, it might go away' / 'If I don't try, I won't fail'. These are understandable attempts to come up with *rules for living* that might make life bearable or make life seem manageable. Sometimes they work, sometimes they work for a short time – but sometimes they backfire. In the first example the man might have such strong fears that he is overwhelmed and so he avoids talking about them. This avoidance, this behaviour, means that he's never able to discover if his fears were founded or not and so his worries and anxiety remain high. In the second example I was initially so pessimistic that I didn't properly explore avenues and talk to others about coping, so there was the danger that I wouldn't learn that there might be ways of dealing with despondency. At these times it's not uncommon to find comfort in the short term by raiding the pantry, taking up smoking again or going on a spending spree, but if that is always our coping strategy we don't learn healthier ways of dealing with distress and, what's more, our real concerns might not be resolved.

By now you can probably see the patterns: the way we feel and think influences what we do and this, in turn, affects how we think and feel. And it's this interaction of thinking, feeling and our behaviour that can create 'traps'.

Faced with the task of having to sort out Udo's complicated taxes at a time when we were stressed by many other worries, the thought in my mind was: 'I can't possibly do this, it's too much.' This type of thought often leads to avoidance, and avoidance means never discovering if we actually can cope. So, the fear and the prediction – 'I can't possibly do that' – remain untested. Fear coupled with avoidance is a common anxiety trap and the tendency is that the more we avoid what frightens us, the more frightening it becomes. I eventually got around to tackling the taxes but not before the task had grown incredibly daunting and was causing me stress that was way out of proportion to the situation.

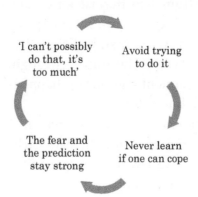

'I can't possibly do that, it's too much'

Avoid trying to do it

The fear and the prediction stay strong

Never learn if one can cope

Here's another trap, a typical depression trap: the thought, 'There's no point,' gives an edge to depression and the behaviour of giving up saps hope.

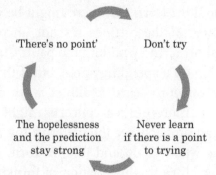

'There's no point'   Don't try

The hopelessness   Never learn
and the prediction   if there is a point
stay strong   to trying

This wasn't something that we saw in Udo; he was remarkably optimistic, but he recalled many patients who were held back in their rehabilitation because of a hopeless state of mind. I frequently found myself in the hopeless trap, but then I've always been something of a pessimist. And that's another relevant point – when we are under stress our natural tendencies can become exaggerated, so the worrier can find themselves overwhelmed with anxieties, the pessimist can be brought very low or the short tempered amongst us can find themselves easily enraged. All of which further fuels 'traps'.

CBT helps us identify these unhelpful patterns and understand where they come from, how they backfire – and ultimately how to break free of them. There are two advantages to appreciating what drives these vicious cycles: first, realising: 'It's no wonder I have these difficulties, look at the trap I'm caught up in,' can be a shame-reducing moment and once it happens, we can consider how we might do things differently.

Second, if we can map out patterns, we can start to predict how our traps unfold and we can anticipate each stage in the trap, which means that we can work out ways of disrupting the patterns and then we can escape them.

Once we've got an understanding of the trap, CBT encourages us to stand back, review and reconsider the negative or unhelpful thoughts that we've identified. When we do this, it is possible to begin to develop new perspectives and new possibilities and CBT then encourages us to try them out, daring to behave differently. This might mean that someone:

- faces their fear in manageable steps, or
- gets increasingly active in the face of hopelessness, or
- turns away from conflict instead of reacting angrily.

In essence, CBT shows us how to break free of old patterns and create new ones – new ways of being that can build confidence and self-worth. Once this happens, we *feel* better in ourselves – and that's the ultimate goal. It's an elegant therapy and in this chapter, I'll share what I hope is a helpful version of it, but before I take you through the practice of CBT, I need to tell you a bit more about my own experience of using it.

I've been a CBT therapist since the 1980s: that's a long time so it's not surprising that I turned to it after my husband's stroke, but it was surprising how hard I had to work at it. Knowing CBT doesn't necessarily translate into effortless application, and sometimes I felt that I'd let the side down because I struggled or, instead of following the line of CBT, I sank my head in the sand or turned to a generous nightcap. CBT did help me, but it was not without effort and I was not spared setbacks and times of despair. One reason for the struggle was that our stresses and challenges kept coming: goalposts kept shifting and fresh disappointments and threats would appear. This must be the reality for many families surviving a stroke; the situation can be one of ongoing adversity. Luckily, CBT is relevant even when the situation really is bad because it's not about convincing yourself that things are okay when they are not; it's about getting a perspective that means that you don't overestimate the downside and you don't underestimate your resources to cope. I often forgot my resources: the friends, family and professionals who could guide us. As a result, I felt more alone and helpless than I needed to, or, as you'll see later, I overestimated how bad or hopeless the situation was.

That said, let's get back to CBT. My aim here is to keep it simple but for those who want more detailed self-help texts, then we've put a list of excellent publications in Chapter 9.

The first and essential step in self-help is identifying your own 'traps'. Try to spot the signs – drinking too much, putting things off too readily, mood getting lower, for example. Each of us has different patterns and you need to be familiar with yours.

Then there are essentially three top tips for breaking free from traps:

- Catch the problem thought/image and step back from it: take stock
- Distract or rethink
- Try out a new way of doing things

This requires us to take a detached stance and to be prepared to risk trying out something new, which is sometimes easier said than done, but it does get easier with familiarity and practice.

Catch the problem thought/ image and step back from it

Catching a thought (or mental image) sounds simple enough, but this can take practice. The tell-tale sign of a troubling thought or image is often a distressing feeling. I remember returning from the hospital in the first weeks following the stroke. Night after night, house dark, kids silent, and I just felt 'bad', I wasn't really aware of thoughts. When I dwelt on this feeling it was very physical: constricted throat, mild nausea and a leadenness in my body. The feeling that came with it can best be described as 'impending doom', a lonely sense of bleak prospects. Focusing on this helped me clarify the thoughts:

- This can't be happening, it isn't fair.
- How can I cope?
- We've lost the man we loved; we've lost the life we had, the hopes and security for the future. It's going to get worse; it keeps getting worse.

There were also two images that kept cropping up and images are very often more emotionally powerful than words, so it is important to look out for them. One of my images was more of what we call a 'flashback', an intense reliving of a moment. It is as if – at least emotionally – we are back at an early scene. My flashback at these times was Udo's face, slightly twisted with vacant eyes, and it captured the moment when I believed that we'd 'lost' the person that he was. The picture was vivid and when it came to mind I was transported back to his bedside, reliving the shock and the loss. The image soon disappeared but it always left me shaken. Flashbacks can be dramatic, but they are also a normal response to extremely emotional situations and, in most instances, they fade over time. Fortunately for me this image faded as the weeks passed and as we had more glimpses of an Udo that we knew.

The second image was not an intense and vivid image, just a fleeting mental picture of an isolated and defeated person, who was me. Despite it being rather shadowy and short-lived it still packed an emotional punch and dragged me down. Unlike the flashback, this image didn't fade over time.

In the early hours of the morning these thoughts and images were even harder to tolerate.

Stepping back from a troubling thought or mental picture has been called 'helicoptering' by a colleague, Dr Melanie Fennell. By this she means mentally detaching and rising above the situation, seeing the trap as a pattern, viewing the thoughts as thoughts and the feelings as feelings, distinguishing the pain of 'now' from the past or future when things were and can again be different. This is sometimes sufficient to break out of the trap. The recognition that a thought is just a thought, a memory is just an image, that things can be different can sometimes give us a new perspective, one that is more manageable.

Sometimes it helps to write down the thought – it captures it on paper and immediately creates a distance.

I wrote down my thoughts and images and also my responses.

Thought / Image	My response
This can't be happening, it isn't fair.	It is happening and it's not fair. I understand why I think like this but there's nothing to be done about it. Oddly enough this thought doesn't bother me so much now I've actually stated it.
How can I cope?	Turn a question into a statement: 'I fear that I can't cope, that emotionally I will be unable to support and protect the kids and Udo. We've no "back-up" parent now so I have to cope. If I don't then they could fall apart, go off the rails, fail their exams, never get a decent job, not have a future.' This scares me – it's a real worry that stays with me.
We've lost the man we loved; we've lost the life we had, the hopes and security for the future. It's going to get worse; it keeps getting worse.	This all seems so true right now. I can't get a different perspective. It drags me down to dwell on it, but the thought keeps coming into my mind.
Image: an isolated and defeated person.	I now realise how powerful this is, particularly in the early hours. I now understand my feelings better.

Having strong feelings triggered by negative thoughts isn't something that is limited to the early days of a crisis. Long after the initial shock of Udo's stroke I'd find myself noticing something lovely and then feeling dreadful. At first it didn't make sense that I felt awful when I realised that I was taking a delightful walk with a friend or noticing the beautiful city we lived in. But I tracked my thinking and discovered a pattern that made sense of my feelings: 'This is lovely . . . I'm lucky that I can enjoy it . . . Udo can't.' Then I'd feel sad, guilty even. Once I could understand why I was distressed by good experiences I could stand back and not be so drawn in by the negative feelings.

Once the problem thoughts or images are defined, it's possible to stand back and when we stand back we often find it easier to deal with them. For example, just writing down the first thought did the trick. The others weren't so simply dealt with but once they were on paper it was easier to take a good look at them.

One of the first things we can do is look for what another colleague, Dr Gillian Butler, calls 'crooked thinking'. Thinking that makes us feel worse because it is:

- **Exaggerated:** perhaps we only see the extremes of a situation or we hold unrealistic standards, or we leap to the very, very worst conclusion.
- **Self-reproachful:** we might be hard on ourselves, perhaps call ourselves names, taking things personally. All of which tends to make a person feel even worse.
- **Skewed to the negative:** perhaps we assume the worst because of one event, or always see the glass 'half empty' or dismiss positive experiences.
- **Based on intuition:** assuming that something must be true because it 'feels' true – so there's no arguing with it. This includes jumping to conclusions or 'mind-reading'.

In my example, I could pick out exaggerated thinking when I scrutinised my worries about the future of my family: 'They could fall apart, go off the rails, fail their exams, never get a decent job, not have a future.' This helped me realise that I was assuming the very, very worst – catastrophising as it's sometimes called. Giving it this label helped me detach a little and took some of the edge off the distress, but it didn't quite fix things because the worries continued to haunt me.

The same was true when I looked at my next thought: 'We've lost the man we loved; we've lost the life we had, the hopes and security for the future. It's going to get worse; it keeps getting worse.' Again, I could see that my thinking was skewed to the negative, only seeing the worst of the situation and predicting even more misery. This is an easy trap to fall into when we are scared and unhappy and realising how exaggerated my thinking had become did help a little but once more the thought still haunted me – as did the exaggerated image of an isolated and defeated person.

I needed strategies to help me to deal with the thoughts and images that just wouldn't go away. This is when learning to distract myself or to rethink the situation eased things for me.

Distract or rethink

Distraction is a standard CBT technique that rests on the fact that none of us can really concentrate on two things at once. Yes, we can pay scant attention to several things but if we actually properly focus on something that is neutral or even pleasant, we can displace upsetting thoughts and images. There is a description of distraction and some examples of distraction techniques in Chapter 9.

Distraction gave me a strategy that I could use to put aside worry. One worry that was particularly troublesome was the concern that I couldn't cope.

Dr Gillian Butler has a beautifully simple guideline for dealing with worries:

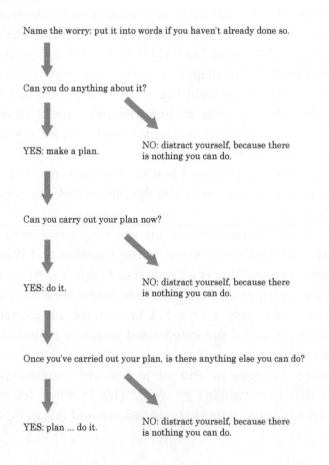

Name the worry: put it into words if you haven't already done so.

Can you do anything about it?

YES: make a plan.

NO: distract yourself, because there is nothing you can do.

Can you carry out your plan now?

YES: do it.

NO: distract yourself, because there is nothing you can do.

Once you've carried out your plan, is there anything else you can do?

YES: plan ... do it.

NO: distract yourself, because there is nothing you can do.

And so on, until you can rest assured that you've done what you can, and you might as well set the worry aside.

I realised that I was doing all that I could to hold things together and worrying was just making it harder to get on with day-to-day pressures. There was nothing more that I could do at this time, so I used distraction to help me park my worries until such time that I could actually resolve some of our difficulties.

I had several distraction strategies as I needed different techniques at different times. At work I might take some time out to illustrate a PowerPoint presentation – I found searching Google Images absorbing, and I felt that I was doing something valid with my time if illustrations made my teaching more memorable. Alternatively, I'd see if a colleague was free to wander over to the hospital café with me. In the car I had a range of soothing and uplifting music, music that I could also listen to at home. But at home there were other things that I could do. When it is particularly hard to distract ourselves, physical activity often works better than mental tasks. So, I would take a walk to the nearby shops rather than jumping into the car or I'd brave the cold and hack at a few shrubs in the garden.

Distraction was definitely my go-to technique in the early hours when it's hard for any of us to think sensibly. I had an iPad by the bed and would often reach for it at 3 a.m. At first, I couldn't be distracted by news programmes (too upsetting) or documentaries (too demanding) and for a week or two I settled for *Homes Under the Hammer*. It was easy on the intellect; the presenters seemed genuinely nice, warm, gentle people to have in the background at 3 a.m., and for some reason lots of the properties were in the Stoke-on-Trent or Crewe area, not far from where I grew up, and this was comforting. As time progressed I graduated to historical documentaries and feel-good films. In fact, I asked friends for recommendations for cheering films and I ended up watching or re-watching: *Pride, The History Boys, The Big Lebowski* and *Withnail and I*. Had Udo chosen the film it would have been *Groundhog Day* while our son would have recommended *Hot Fuzz* and his sister the musical *Cats*.

A number of books will suggest that, if you can't sleep, you should get up and do something else rather than use the bed for anything but sleep or sex. I would suggest that you experiment and find out what works for you in those early days. For me, *Homes Under the Hammer* was better than getting up or any sleeping draught – each programme lasted less than half an hour and I never saw one to the end because I was fast asleep within minutes. Later, when life had settled, I found that I could get myself back to sleep more naturally, usually by redirecting my thoughts to soothing images. So, I was able to resume a sleep regime more in line with the recommendations of sleep experts.

As time went on, our circumstances did change; I began to adapt to our new situation, and I felt less overwhelmed. I found that I used distraction less and less to manage troubling thoughts and images. I was able to work out something that I could do about immediate problems or I could review them and get a more helpful perspective. This was an important step forward as distraction can backfire if we use it to avoid facing challenges that we could rise to. I had used distraction to deal with my thoughts about the loss of 'Udo' and our future. For a while this worked. Setting aside my concerns gave me some respite and, to be honest, I didn't have the emotional resources to tackle them head-on in those early days. So, I kept using distraction. However, the thoughts returned, especially when I was fatigued. After several weeks of not being able to shake them off and having had some time to adjust to our new situation, I found that I could face my concerns more directly.

The approach that CBT suggests is catching the thought, considering why it makes sense that you think like this, then reviewing what might conflict with your conclusion – all this enables you to rethink it and perhaps get a more helpful perspective.

My recurrent concerns were reflected in three thoughts and I tackled them one at a time.

Thought / Image	It's no wonder I think this . . .	. . . on the other hand . . .	Rethink the thought
We've lost the man we loved.	I look at Udo and it's not him. His gaze is often vacant, and he doesn't think and speak like the Udo I knew.	Staff members are still saying 'early days' so there is time for change, and I do see glimpses of old 'Udo' from time to time.	I'm jumping to conclusions too soon. It is hard going but there is still hope.
We've lost the life we had, the hopes and security for the future.	This is true: we no longer have the security, the freedoms and the opportunities that we had before the stroke.	There is time for things to improve, even if it's not full recovery. And even if we don't get our old life back we can probably still manage, life will just be different.	I'm jumping to conclusions too soon. There is still hope and we might be able to cope even if Udo remains disabled.
It's going to get worse; it keeps getting worse.	It does seem to get worse – infections set in and I can't see much improvement.	Infections can slow progress. I see Udo every day, so it is hard to notice progress.	I'm catastrophising. I should give it time, let Udo recover from setbacks and remember that the signs of recovery can be subtle.

Thinking of the worst fear can be hard, but if we can name it there is more of a chance that we can generate ways of coping. My fear was that Udo would remain disabled physically and cognitively and this would mean significant changes in the immediate future. For example, losing my partner and our children losing their father, his having to move to a care home, having to sell the house (our home – the one stable thing in our lives right now), and so on. Facing the fear meant that I could scrutinise it and see that I was catastrophising (yet again) and I could appreciate that there were things I could do, such as talking with the professionals who might help me develop a realistic view of prognosis, seeking financial advice, lowering my stress by saying no to new projects and asking for extensions on work that was due in. This helped. I didn't feel great, but I was more able to cope.

I was still left with the fleeting but distressing image, though. I could understand why I had it: I did feel alone and overwhelmed by events. I could try to take the sting out of it by reminding myself that '. . . on the other hand there are people to support us', but dealing with an upsetting mental picture is often best done through imagery. By that I mean changing the impact of the image by visualising something more tolerable. Sometimes people find that visually shrinking the image takes the power out of it, or they imagine it on a TV screen and mute the sound or dim the colours in order to reduce the emotional impact. You need to work out what works for you. My image was bleak and dark, and the figure was huddled, but I found that if I allowed sunlight to flood the room and imagined the figure standing strong I could stop it being so distressing. If I then 'saw' the figure walking tall and exiting the room I could dismiss the image and get on with things, at least for a while. At night when the image was harder to deal with I 'saw' the strong figure of myself walking to our two children and enfolding them in my arms, and this gave me a warm feeling and a sense of hope that we'd get through. I practised and practised this soothing image until it came to mind very easily and quite quickly displaced the disturbing image of myself.

All this took hard work – negative thoughts and images often put up quite a fight, but I usually found that I was able to take the edge off fear and hopelessness and sadness and this was enough to keep going. Nonetheless, I found that, even two years on, our waking thoughts were still often about the stroke – 'If only . . .' and 'What if . . .' – and, at bedtime, bad memories and troublesome images still intruded. So, managing the thoughts is an ongoing task.

Try out a new way of doing things

Sometimes we need to follow up on our thinking by *doing*. This means that we test out our new conclusions. There are essentially two ways of doing this:

- By talking it through with someone
- By actively doing something differently

For me, daring to do something differently often meant taking my head out of the sand and confronting a fear or a challenge. As I've already said, I found that a lot of administration follows a stroke: getting sick certificates, informing employers of health status, applying for permission to modify the house, completing documents for claiming sick pay and disability allowances, paying spouse's bills, and so on and so on. I have always disliked admin and my inclination was to put things off – just for a little while – because I felt so overwhelmed, but this took me straight into the procrastination trap.

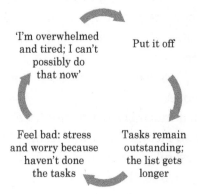

'I'm overwhelmed and tired; I can't possibly do that now'

Put it off

Tasks remain outstanding; the list gets longer

Feel bad: stress and worry because haven't done the tasks

I could review my thoughts and come up with the conclusion that it was understandable that I put off tasks given that I was tired, trying to hold down a job and support the kids and so on, but it was clear that procrastination just made me more stressed and less able to take on the dreaded paperwork. I'd probably feel and function better if I got down to completing the forms and collating the necessary information. At this point, my conclusion is little more than a hunch, a hypothesis – and I don't actually feel any better now that I've developed it; in fact, I feel worse because it's so obvious what I should be doing that I feel foolish for not doing it!

Clearly, I need to change my behaviour to break out of the trap but the thought of all that paperwork is off-putting. This is where breaking down the task into smaller steps pays off. I worked out what I could delegate and what needed to be done most urgently. I then started to check off the tasks according to urgency – often only keeping just ahead of deadlines but I had a strategy that took me out of the trap of falling back further and further. I didn't manage to do this overnight – it took rather longer than that – but it eased the stress and the next application form or bill or letter from the taxman didn't send me straight into 'ostrich mode'.

Another trap that I fell into was the withdrawing into myself, which meant that I probably didn't seek advice as much as I might have and that brought me down and made me more inclined to withdraw. Thus, my concerns and worries would often go untested and that's not good. Take the rethinking that I'd done about our lost life – I'd reached a comforting conclusion: 'There is still hope and we might be able to cope even if Udo remains disabled.' But in order to feel more confident I needed to get some support for my new thought. I needed to turn to people and check out their views and experiences.

When I did, I felt much better because friends and staff shared stories of coping and I learnt that it was realistic to hang on to hope at this stage. So, a useful question to ask yourself when you've developed a new conclusion is: 'How can I check this out?' This really captures the essence of *cognitive behavioural* therapy. Revise the *way you think* and revise *what you do* so that you break free from traps and develop new ways of being that ultimately help you feel better.

There are just a couple more things that it might be useful to say about CBT: it advocates keeping the positive in mind (but only realistically so) and it advocates getting active.

Keeping the positives in mind

When we are in a fragile state of mind, it's too easy to see the negatives in life and to have a 'blindsight' for good things, especially as there seems to be no time for emotional recovery if you are struggling with ongoing disability. It can sometimes seem as if we are stuck in a negative mindset.

As far back as the 1970s, research has shown us that our current state of mind colours how we interpret our world and how we remember our lives. So, when we are in a good mood we tend to recall times when life was good, and we tend to see the world around us as manageable, but if we are down or anxious, our recollections are skewed towards sad or anxious memories and we perceive our current lives negatively: it's as if a 'negative lens' is in place that colours our view. And this can take us straight into another trap.

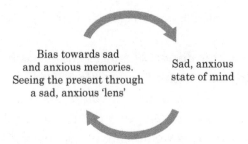

Bias towards sad and anxious memories. Seeing the present through a sad, anxious 'lens'

Sad, anxious state of mind

In order to break out of this pattern of negative thinking and feeling we need to take our thinking to a more positive place. A starting point is making efforts to appreciate the positive things we still have – even the smallest things like a view into a garden, the smell of blossoms as spring comes around, giggling over an episode of *Doctor Who* on Dad's laptop. But when we are not in a good frame of mind it is really easy to forget the good things that are happening so it's wise to jot them down and keep a log of the positives in life. I kept one at the back of the daily journal that I wrote for the first eighteen months after Udo's stroke. The entries varied enormously, some seeming quite insignificant and others seeming much more important, but they all went down in the record because each one raised a smile. Here are just a few:

- Condolences cards from Udo's colleagues and patients all saying how highly they regarded him
- Our son getting a Duke of Edinburgh Award
- Our daughter winning the school poetry prize (although it was a very bleak poem!)
- A Christmas tree brought into Udo's hospital room by friends
- The sunsets across the car park at Udo's hospital
- Smartphone still working after being dropped down the loo
- Udo no longer needing a quad stick for walking
- Another delicious fish pie / rice pudding (from neighbours) on the doorstep
- A birthday gathering of good friends who really made the effort for Udo
- Udo being invited to join a research team

Over time there were dozens of entries and it was helpful to look over them purely as a reminder that life was still balanced – this would help to break free of the trap of biased thinking. Also, by keeping this record we developed a talent, the knack for looking out for the positive. This would help protect us against automatically thinking negatively.

Getting the most out of dwelling on the positive can be heightened by developing the skill of mindfulness. This refers to a state of mind and level of concentration sometimes called 'thought watching' and it can be likened to meditation. So, if I were to be mindful in appreciating the sunset across the car park, rather than just noting it and taking some brief pleasure from it, I might sit in the car, relax and truly savour the moment, observing the play of the light across the clouds and the sounds in the air, detaching from worries or tensions, completely free of self-judgement. Mindfulness is an area of psychology that has been very well researched and successfully combined with CBT (mindful-ness-based cognitive therapy: MBCT). MBCT in particular has been rigorously evaluated and for years now we have known that people who can achieve a meditative state of calm detachment tend to be less vulnerable to depression and anxieties. So, it might be worth considering investing in training.

There are now many good books describing mindfulness train-ing and there are specialist therapists throughout the country. Proper mindful meditation is something that demands a good deal of practice and I have to admit that I have never managed to achieve the deeper levels of detachment that would be the goal of training. This does not mean that mindfulness training wasn't for me; it's just that I got the timing wrong. When I attended courses some years ago, I was caring for two small children and at work I was carrying a full caseload and other responsibilities, so I found it difficult to find time to practise the exercises between classes and I was exhausted. Perhaps not surprisingly, in each of the classes I tended to drift into sleep when we lay on blankets and beanbags and relaxed. At some point a kindly person would nudge me and I'd come to my senses like the dormouse in *Alice in Wonderland* – a bit disorientated and embarrassed. So, timing is important – right now might be a good time to consider train-ing or you might be better off leaving it for a while. Meanwhile, you could still try to savour the moment when things go well, really appreciating how it feels when something is pleasing, rather than just noting it as an event for your 'Positives Record'.

Another research finding is that people recover better from trauma (and having a stroke is a trauma for both the patient and the family) if they look to the past to put their distress into context but then really focus their energies on looking to the future, envisaging how they can now best live life.

I know that I fell into the habit of over-reviewing the past – retelling our story over and over again, getting stuck in a rut of recollection. In the early days this was an important aspect of dealing with our distress, it was an emotional 'working through' the shock of events, it was part of a necessary grieving process. But eventually it turned into something that wasn't helpful; in fact, it dragged me down. I had some notion that analysing our crisis would somehow help us find solutions. At first this might have been the case but weeks and months later it just reminded me of a sad situation, and I felt worse. My mood only began to lift as I started to get on top of tasks and plan for a new future, even if it was a future that we hadn't wanted.

Reviewing the past for Udo was quite a different thing. In the first few months following his stroke, he'd lived in the past but rather than thinking of the time of his brain bleed, his recollections were of his earlier, happiest times and for a while this buoyed him up, so it was a constructive state of mind. However, when it started to hold him back from preparing for the future, it was far from helpful.

Another trap that it's easy to fall into is idealising the lost future, imagining the happiness and security that might have been. While this initially might be an important aspect of grieving, repeatedly reviewing the future that we've lost can bring us down – and anyway, who knows if our fantasy future was realistic?

Getting active

There are two reasons for getting active: as we've seen, it is an important way of checking out our beliefs, be they the old way of thinking or new theories. Another reason for getting active is that research shows us that being inactive can worsen our problems. If we are anxious then a common inactivity is avoidance and when we are depressed a common inactivity is withdrawing from social and work commitments. The two cycles below show how these traps work.

Avoidance of the things that we fear stops us from learning that we can do something, so we stay anxious; withdrawal robs us of positive feedback from our friends or our work and that fuels depression.

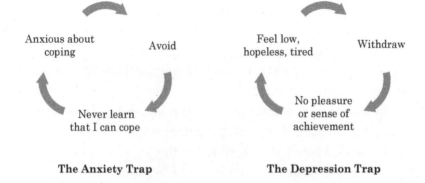

The Anxiety Trap   **The Depression Trap**

Udo grew nervous about being in the street in his wheelchair. He felt vulnerable and he was scared that I might topple the chair on the uneven pavements and that he might fall and have another head injury or worse. So he asked not to be taken for outings to the local shops. We stopped going out and his confidence just got worse and worse.

I felt low-spirited initially and just closed in on myself. I turned down social invitations and so I had fewer uplifting outings and I had more time to ruminate on how difficult things were and this made me more low-spirited and even less inclined to engage in social activities.

The only way to overcome anxiety is to face the fear. If this seems too much to tackle head-on, then break the task down into small steps. We planned Udo's outings so that we first took a very safe route just around the hospital grounds where the pavement surface was quite good and there were well-positioned dropped kerbs. When he was relaxed about that journey we ventured further afield but still planned routes where the pavement was smooth and there were few junctions to be negotiated. Eventually we dared to go to the local shops via back streets with the most atrocious surfaces that forced me to leave the pavement altogether and push the chair on the road. This was not something that we wanted to repeat but we learnt that even on really bad surfaces and narrow pavements Udo could be safe.

As you might have worked out for yourself, overcoming depression that is fuelled by inactivity requires us to become active. Not only does this break the cycle by increasing the chance of getting pleasure or a sense of achievement but we also know that exercise alone improves mood. Plenty of research shows this to be the case so it is another good reason to get active. I began to increase the activities that the kids and I did together, so we were less likely just to retreat to our own parts of the house when we were at home. We found films to watch together and I tried to instigate a regular walk. I rarely managed to get the kids to join me on the walk but at least it got me active. And I began to say yes to social invitations. Some people find that they are helped by seeing groups of friends, but it was months before I could face anything more than one or two at a time. In the early days, Udo didn't get caught up in a depression trap thanks to regular visitors and the daily positive feedback that he got from staff who encouraged him in rehabilitation. It was only when he got home and the social interactions and the positive feedback and the intensity of exercise diminished that he seemed to get low in his spirits. Fortunately, by then I was feeling more upbeat and had the energy to enforce outings, invite people over and encourage him to do his physical exercises.

Relatively recent research has shown us that purposeful, not just pleasurable, activities can improve our mood. So, it's not just the fun things but the meaningful things – the activities that make us feel as though we've done something worthwhile – that lift our spirits. When at last we were able to take a holiday and visit family in Germany, we certainly enjoyed binge-viewing DVDs (and it was good to do this as a family) but we achieved a more lasting sense of contentment after we'd taken a long walk to find some of Udo's favourite German foods and I felt uplifted after I'd worked on this book for an hour or so, even though it might have initially been a less inviting prospect than the DVDs.

I'm used to making a mental note of how pleasurable or purposeful (or satisfying) I find things but if you aren't, it can be helpful to keep a detailed log (so that you can review what gives you pleasure and satisfaction) until it starts to become second nature. Below is an example of a couple of days of diary keeping where I use a 1/10 – 10/10 rating scale where 1 represents no pleasure or purposefulness/ satisfaction and 10 represents maximum pleasure or purposefulness/ satisfaction.

	Monday	Tuesday
6.00–7.00	Lying awake, beginning to worry about various things Pleasure (P): 1/10 **(No pleasure)** Sense of purposefulness, satisfaction (PS): 1/10 **(No purposefulness / satisfaction)**	Begin marking essays with pot of fresh coffee to hand P: 5/10 PS: 9/10
7.00–9.00	The usual washing, dressing and breakfasting routine with Udo P: 4/10 **(Neutral)** PS 8/10 **(Satisfying)**	The usual washing, dressing and breakfasting routine with Udo P: 5/10 PS: 8/10
9.00–10.00	General household chores P: 3/10 PS: 6/10	Essay marking P: 6/10 PS: 9/10
10.00–11.00	Joining in Udo's physiotherapy session P: 8/10 PS: 8/10	
11.00	Nip out to local shops alone P: 2/10 PS: 7/10	Take a break: coffee and cake with Udo P: 8/10 PS: 8/10
11.00–12.30		Back to marking essays while Udo works alone on his physical exercises P: 5/10 PS: 8/10
12.30–1.00	Lunch with Udo P: 8/10 PS: 6/10	
1.00–2.00	Sorting out pension issues and other necessary 'paperwork' P: 3/10 PS 9/10	Drive to hospital for Udo's clinic appointments (lunch in car). Sit in hospital café working on book while I wait P: 7/10 PS: 9/10
2.00–3.00		
3.00–4.00	Friend for tea P: 9/10 PS: 7/10	
4.00–5.00		Drive home via supermarket. Udo waits in car P: 2/10 PS: 7/10
5.00–6.00	More 'paperwork' P: 3/10 PS: 9/10	

6.00–7.00	Prepare supper, put in some laundry, usual evening chores P: 3/10 PS: 7/10	Direct the kids to the microwave and leave them to get supper: meet friend and colleague in town for a catch–up P: 9/10 PS: 6/10
7.00–8.00 8.00–9.00	Take our son to Scouts and wait for him in local pub (with Udo) P: 9/10 PS: 9/10	
9.00–11.00	The usual evening routine: helping Udo get ready for bed P: 5/10 PS: 8/10	The usual evening routine: helping Udo get ready for bed P: 5/10 PS: 8/10

From this diary, it is easy to see that lying in bed worrying at 6 a.m. is of little value and the time is better spent doing something productive – in my case I made a start on a set of essays that needed marking. It is also obvious that there are many things that are not pleasurable, but if I engaged in them I found them satisfying (for example: getting through paperwork and necessary chores). So, I could use this to remind myself that it is worth facing unattractive tasks because the pay-off is quite significant. I could also see from this diary that, in general, I enjoyed doing things with Udo more than not. So maybe I would stop doing the shopping without him just because it seems convenient at the time – perhaps I could find out if he'd prefer to join me.

Coping with setbacks and lapses

CBT isn't a vaccination against negative thoughts and feelings and from time to time there will be setbacks. You might as well expect them. My cognitive and emotional lapses tended to happen when I was exhausted and/or when a new crisis reared its head. The key to recovering as quickly as you can is to ask yourself three questions:

- Why is it understandable that I've had this setback?
- What have I learnt from it?
- What will I now do differently?

Answering the first question will put you in a compassionate, rather than self-blaming, frame of mind and it will help you pinpoint a reason for the setback. The other two questions will guide you towards problem solving, whereby you learn from setbacks and use that learning to take you forward and make you stronger.

I had such a setback when we heard some very worrying news about my mother's health, and it was understandable that this overloaded my capacity to cope. I learnt that I needed to ensure that I had emotional reserves so that I could manage better and support the family at such times. With hindsight I would have made sure that I had been taking some time out to recharge my batteries. So, I immediately set up some social events with people I knew were warm, supportive and who could be light hearted. But I also had a setback when I simply pranged our new car. It was understandable that I'd bashed it into a bollard – it was in a blind spot and I was preoccupied with getting to the next appointment and was generally quite stressed. Objectively this was not a big deal, nothing like the worry about my mother, yet it set me back – why? Again, it was predominantly because I didn't have much in the way of emotional reserves and it was a real reminder to revive my plans to recharge the batteries.

The point of these examples is to illustrate that we sometimes lapse because of life events that would universally be considered crises but equally we can lapse because that 'last straw' has been placed on our backs. Try to understand that this can trigger a setback rather than beating yourself up for getting upset over something relatively trivial.

I have to be honest and say that I couldn't always stick strictly to the CBT way. There were times when I knew that it was in my best interest to get active but still I lay in bed ruminating and there were times when I knew that it was in my best interest not to put off doing something, yet I did. But that's human and the best way forward is to stand back and be understanding and constructive. So, I might well say to myself:

It is understandable that I couldn't face doing that task, I've been pushing myself hard and I'm exhausted.

However, I know that it's just going to get harder if I leave it for much longer.

Therefore, this is what I'll do: right now, I'll recharge my batteries by taking some time out but tomorrow I will take on the task – but I'll break it down into smaller steps and take it one step at a time so that it doesn't feel so daunting. I'll also discuss it with a colleague and find out how she tackled something similar – perhaps I can learn some tips from her.

This type of review of the situation can help us get back on track without undermining our confidence or our hope. And in the weeks, months and even years following a stroke there will be lots of getting back on track.

Finally

This has been a lengthy chapter – but to be fair, there is a lot to say about CBT and that's why I've recommended some further reading in Chapter 9 for those of you who want to learn more.

We found that our knowledge of CBT helped us, along with the support that we had from family, friends and professionals, and we very much hope that – when the time is right for you – you can use the approach of standing back and reviewing your thinking and revising your behaviours to help you through the difficult times. We hope that this, in turn, gives you more hope and resilience in the times ahead. But remember that we are all different, so some people will find CBT harder to put into practice than others and some might find that it's not for them at all or at least not for a while.

Human beings sit along a spectrum ranging from those who have always been quite resilient and able to appreciate the positive through to those who struggle to keep cheerful. And at different times we can sit at different points on the spectrum. Before Udo's stroke, things were good for us: the kids seemed to be settled, we were getting along better than ever, we were secure and reasonably relaxed, and I would have placed myself nearer the positive end of the spectrum, reasonably resilient and able to deal with the odd crisis and setback (probably using simple CBT techniques without much difficulty). Six months after the stroke, I was in quite a different place, my resilience sapped by relentless worry, huge uncertainty, witnessing the kids' struggles, and of course lack of sleep. I was much nearer the negative end of the spectrum and I needed more support and I had to work harder to keep going than I would have a few months earlier.

For the more resilient amongst us, reading about CBT approaches can be enough to nudge us forward but the less resilient will have to work harder at putting the theory into practice and discovering benefits, and yet others might need some extra support from a counsellor or CBT therapist. If you think that you need additional support don't hold back: speak with your family doctor or hospital staff and see if you can get extra support through the NHS. Alternatively, consider private counselling or private CBT but do check that your therapist is properly trained.

Don't give up; things do tend to get easier. In the Epilogue of this book you'll see that after a two-year period that seemed to drag on so slowly we did see improvement and we did recognise achievements. Admittedly, we'd had to lower our expectations and revise our hopes along the way, and this is where CBT often comes into its own, helping us to keep a realistic perspective.

8

Epilogue

'My husband's mantra of "bit by bit" alongside all the skill and encouragement of the O.C.E. . . . . has meant that seven years post-stroke we are both able to greet each morning with joy.'

Following his stroke, Udo became an outpatient in the O.C.E. Spasticity Clinic. His own spasticity (clonus) was pretty severe and the sometimes violent shaking of his leg stopped him from walking properly and made him fearful of falling. So, he definitely needed Botox injections to his calf muscles.

As we said earlier in the book, Udo had actually set up the Spasticity Clinic at the O.C.E. and for nearly two decades he helped innumerable people gain relief from painful or shaking and constricted muscles. Now the proficient staff that he had supported and trained were there for him. As usual, the quality of medical care was excellent, but the care went much further. Since his stroke, patients attending the clinic had asked after him and many had wanted to pass on their good wishes, so the clinic staff had gone to the trouble of setting up a greetings book for Udo.

They felt we should know just how patients felt about the 'Dear Professor'. So, on one visit he was presented with a notebook bursting with warm wishes. It was incredibly moving to read the comments and we wept as we leafed through the book in the hospital café later. We must have *both* looked very post-stroke with our obvious emotional incontinence.

Some patients added a mini-progress report to their greetings. So we read of continued recovery – for example, people regaining

the ability to speak, successful career changes, improved mobility
– and we were reminded that the brain is indeed plastic and that
continuing to push with rehabilitation can lead to very positive
change.

One particularly encouraging comment came from the wife of
a patient who'd had a stroke seven years earlier and you can see
her statement at the start of this chapter. Recovery can go beyond
moving more, speaking better, thinking more clearly: it is possible to reach a state that even transcends acceptance. This woman
was able to speak of joy, and in the darker moments of recovery it
might be helpful to think on her words.

We stopped writing this book on the two-year anniversary of
Udo's stroke. As we said before, some families get back on track
within months, others within years. For us it felt as though we'd
taken two years to claw back something of a life worth living,
although it is still very much a work in progress. Udo now had
regular meetings with Headway staff and he had set up more
meetings with researchers at both the University of Oxford and
Oxford Brookes University. A meaningful routine was beginning
to emerge to give more shape to his week and the sense of being
worthwhile grew. He was glad to be alive, to be at home and to be
a part of a family. Even so, he felt that he was still grieving, and he
walked a thin line between mourning the loss of his previous life
and abilities and looking forward.

Helen had put many activities on hold following Udo's stroke,
but it now felt like the right time to resume writing commitments
and take on a full clinical caseload again. Our children were now
more at ease and even playful with their dad. The shock and fear
of the first year had lifted and we could see an existence ahead for
them. Our daughter had grown into a woman and was now set to
develop her own life and career and our son had begun his A
levels, with, we hoped, more confidence and stability than he'd
had during the past two years.

On 9 October 2018, exactly two years after the bleed began deep
in Udo's brain, he took a telephone call from a representative of the

National Headway charity congratulating him on being short-listed for the 'Outstanding Contribution to Headway Award'. His years of work were being recognised and he was reminded that he had, and might continue to have, a relevant role in neuro-rehabilitation.

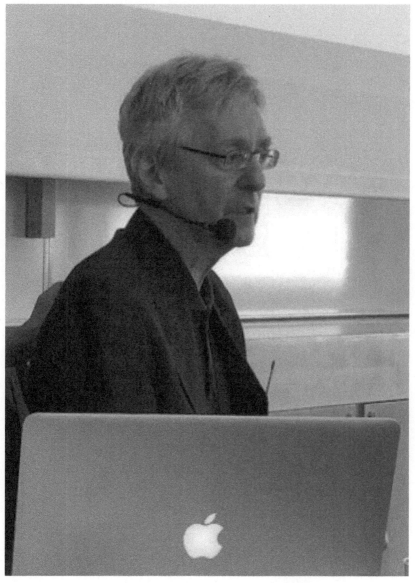

'Professor Kischka' giving a talk in Stockholm

9

Some Useful Resources

This final section of the book comprises some practical additions that you might find useful, namely:

1. A helpful reading list. These are mostly CBT texts but there is one called *Head Injury (The Facts)* that is an excellent short book about understanding and recovering from head injury – and Udo is one of the authors.
2. Key societies and organisations.
3. Additional notes on Relaxation and Distraction to supplement the CBT chapter.
4. Some templates for keeping notes if you want to try out some of the suggestions in the CBT chapter.

Helpful Reading List

Bolte Taylor J., 'My Stroke of Insight' (TED Talk), (www.youtube.com/watch?r=UyyjU8fzEYU, 2008)

Butler G., Grey N. & Hope T., *Manage Your Mind: The mental fitness guide* (OUP, 2017)

Daisley A., Tams R. & Kischka U., *Head Injury (The Facts)* (OUP, 2008)

Espie C., *Overcoming Insomnia and Sleep Problems: A self-help guide to using cognitive behavioural techniques* (Robinson, 2012)

Freeston M. & Meares K., *Overcoming Worry: A self-help guide using cognitive behavioural techniques* (Robinson, 2015)

Gilbert P., *Overcoming Depression: A self-help guide using cognitive behavioural techniques* (Robinson, 2009)

Greenberger D. & Padesky C., *Mind Over Mood: Change how you feel by changing the way you think* (Guilford Press, 2015)

Kennerley H., *Overcoming Anxiety: A self-help guide using cognitive behavioural techniques* (Robinson, 2014)

King N., *Overcoming Mild Traumatic Brain Injury: A self-help guide using evidence-based techniques* (Robinson, 2015)

McCrum R., *My Year Off: Rediscovering life after a stroke)* (Picador, 1998)

Myles P. & Shafran R., *The CBT Handbook: A comprehensive guide to using CBT to overcome depression, anxiety and anger* (Robinson, 2015)

Pratchett T. & Gaiman N., *A Slip of the Keyboard: Collected non-fiction* (Corgi, 2015)

Key Societies and Organisations

The ARNI Institute

An organisation with a physically active approach to stroke recovery with over 100 professional trainers around the UK. www.arni.uk.com

BASIC

Brain and Spinal Injury Centre. A Manchester-based organisation that provides counselling, information and support services for patients and families following a brain or spinal injury. www.basiccharity.org.uk

British Heart Foundation

Provides useful and practical information about stroke and life after stroke. www.bhf.org.uk/informationsupport/conditions/stroke

Carers Trust

A major charity for carers, improving the support needed for those living with a family member who is disabled in some way. www.carers.org

Chest, Heart and Stroke N. Ireland

A charity aimed at improving the quality of life for people in Northern Ireland who have suffered stroke (and some other conditions). www.nichs.org.uk

Chest, Heart and Stroke Scotland

A charity aimed at improving the quality of life for people in Scotland who have suffered stroke (and some other conditions). www.chss.org.uk

Different strokes

Offers support for the younger stroke survivor and children throughout the UK. www.differentstrokes.co.uk

Headway: the brain injury association

A national charity that promotes understanding of all aspects of brain injury and provides information, support and services to survivors, their families and carers. There are many local branches nationwide. www.headway.org.uk

NHS Choices Stroke website

A regularly updated website that clearly defines stroke and documents key aspects of treatment and recovery, including getting social support and care. www.nhs.uk/conditions/stroke

The Stroke Association

One of the leading UK charities dedicated to supporting stroke survivors and their families and investing in stroke research and education. www.stroke.org.uk

Relaxation and Distraction

Relaxation training

This is an invaluable self-help skill and one that is relatively easy to learn, but it does require practice.

The skill of relaxing is different from simply using activities like curling up with a book or watching TV to relax. We all need to have a repertoire of relaxing things that we do but in addition we can learn how to relax at will, turning on the relaxation response whenever we are aware that we feel tense. Just as learning a language or learning an instrument is a structured task that takes time and practice, so does the skill of relaxation. Below is a set of exercises that, if rehearsed regularly, will enable you to combat tension whenever you need to.

Some people find it helpful to make a recording of the instructions. We have provided recordings for your use at www.overcoming.co.uk/715/resources-to-download but the full scripts are provided below if you prefer to record your own. If you do, then you will want to make as soothing a recording as possible, so choose a time when you are feeling reasonably relaxed and your voice is not strained, and you are not hurried.

As a regular breathing pattern is fundamental to achieving a relaxed state, it's a good idea to begin with getting this right.

Preliminary regular breathing

INSTRUCTIONS:
Find a comfortable position and let your body grow heavy.

*Attend to your breathing for a moment just allowing this to be as
    natural as possible.*
*Try to breathe through your nose if you can, making your breath-
    ing smooth and even.*
*On the next out-breath try to empty your lungs, right down to your
    diaphragm – as if you were breathing from your stomach.*
Take a gentle in-breath counting slowly to five: one, two, three, four, five.
*Imagine filling your lungs completely, right down to your
    diaphragm.*
Breathe out slowly: one, two, three, four, five, six.
Imagine emptying your lungs.
Breathe in: one, two, three, four, five.
Breathe out slowly: one, two, three, four, five, six.
Breathe in: one, two, three, four, five.
Breathe out slowly: one, two, three, four, five, six.
Try to keep this pattern during your relaxation exercises.

Deep Relaxation Exercise

Now you can move on to a thorough relaxation exercise that helps us
distinguish between muscular tension and relaxation whilst instruct-
ing us to relax at will. It is particularly useful when we are so used to
being tense that we find it difficult even to appreciate that we are
tense. It is also an excellent exercise for those of us who struggle to
let go of tension in the muscles or who need a step-by-step training
because we are so unfamiliar with the sensations of relaxation. The
procedure involves working through various muscle groups first
tensing and then relaxing them. The exercises start with the feet,
working up through the body slowly and smoothly, letting the sensation of relaxation deepen at its own pace. However, if you'd rather
start elsewhere in the body it's fine to do so. You need to try out the
exercises and adapt them so that they work for you.

   You will need to tense your muscles – but do not to overdo this.
The aim is to tighten muscles but not to strain. No one should get
pain or cramps!

INSTRUCTIONS:

First, get as comfortable as you can . . . Lie flat on the floor with a pillow under your head, or snuggle in your chair . . . If you wear glasses, remove them . . . Kick off your shoes and loosen any tight clothing . . . Relax your arms by your sides and have your legs uncrossed. Close your eyes, and don't worry if they flicker – this is quite usual. Don't worry if random thoughts enter your mind – this is also quite usual. Just let them go and then refocus on relaxing.

You are beginning to relax . . . Breathe out slowly . . . Now, breathe in smoothly and deeply . . . Now, breathe out slowly again, imagining yourself becoming heavier and heavier, sinking into the floor (or your chair) . . . Keep breathing rhythmically, and feel a sense of relief and of letting go . . . Try saying 'relax' to yourself as you breathe out . . . Breathe like this for a few moments more . . .

Now, begin to tense and relax the muscles of your body . . . Think of your feet . . . Tense the muscles in your feet and ankles, curling your toes towards your head . . . Gently stretch your muscles . . . Feel the tension in your feet and ankles . . . Hold it . . . Now let go . . . Let your feet go limp and floppy . . . Feel the difference . . . Feel the tension draining away from your feet . . . Let your feet roll outwards and grow heavier and heavier . . . Imagine that they are so heavy that they are sinking into the floor . . . More and more relaxed . . . Growing heavier and more relaxed . . . (REPEAT)

Now, think about your calves . . . Begin to tense the muscles in your lower legs . . . If you are sitting, lift your legs up and hold them in front of you, feeling the tension . . . Gently stretch the muscles . . . Feel that tension . . . Hold it . . . Now release . . . Let your feet touch the floor and let your legs go floppy and heavy . . . Feel the difference . . . Feel the tension leaving your legs, draining away from your calves . . . Leaving your calves feeling heavy . . . Draining away from your feet . . . Leaving them feeling heavy and limp . . . Imagine that your legs and feet are so heavy that they are sinking into the floor . . . They feel

*limp and relaxed . . . Growing more and more heavy and
relaxed . . . (REPEAT)*

*Think about your thigh muscles . . . Tense them by pushing the
tops of your legs together as hard as you can . . . Feel the tension
building . . . Hold it . . . Now, let your legs fall apart . . . Feel the
difference . . . Feel the tension draining away from your legs . . .
They feel limp and heavy . . . Your thighs feel heavy . . . Your
calves feel heavy . . . Your feet feel heavy . . . Imagine the tension
draining away . . . Leaving your legs . . . Leaving them feeling
limp and relaxed . . . Leaving them feeling so heavy that they
are sinking into the floor or your chair . . . Let the feelings of
relaxation spread up from your feet . . . Up through your
legs . . . Relaxing your hips and lower back . . . (REPEAT)*

*Now tense the muscles of your hips and lower back by squeezing
your buttocks together . . . Arch your back, gently . . . Feel the
tension . . . Hold the tension . . . Now let it go . . . Let your
muscles relax . . . Feel your spine supported again . . . Feel the
muscles relax . . . Deeper and deeper . . . More and more
relaxed . . . Growing heavier and heavier . . . Your hips are
relaxed . . . Your legs are relaxed . . . Your feet are heavy . . .
Tension is draining away from your body . . . (REPEAT)*

*Tense your stomach and chest muscles; imagine that you are
expecting a punch in the stomach and prepare yourself for the
impact . . . Take in a breath, and as you do, pull in your stomach and feel the muscles tighten . . . Feel your chest muscles
tighten and become rigid . . . Hold the tension . . . Now slowly
breathe out and let go of the tension . . . Feel your stomach
muscles relax . . . Feel the tightness leave your chest . . . As you
breathe evenly and calmly, your chest and stomach should
gently rise and fall . . . Allow your breathing to become rhythmic
and relaxed . . . (REPEAT)*

*Now think about your hands and arms . . . Slowly curl your fingers
into two tight fists . . . Feel the tension . . . Now hold your arms
straight out in front of you, still clenching your fists . . . Feel the
tension in your hands, your forearms and your upper arms . . .*

*Hold it . . . Now, let go . . . Gently drop your arms by your side
and imagine the tension draining away from your arms . . .
Leaving your upper arms . . . Leaving your forearms . . .
Draining away from your hands . . . Your arms feel heavy and
floppy . . . Your arms feel limp and relaxed . . . (REPEAT)*
Think about the muscles in your shoulders . . . Tense them by
drawing up your shoulders towards your ears and pull them in
towards your spine . . . Feel the tension across your shoulders
and in your neck . . . Tense the muscles in your neck further by
tipping your head back slightly . . . Hold the tension . . . Now
relax . . . Let your head drop forward . . . Let your shoulders
drop . . . Let them drop even further . . . Feel the tension easing
away from your neck and shoulders . . . Feel your muscles relaxing more and more deeply . . . Your neck is limp, and your
shoulders feel heavy . . . (REPEAT)
Think about your face muscles . . . Focus on the muscles running
across your forehead . . . Tense them by frowning as hard as you
can . . . Hold that tension and focus on your jaw muscles . . .
Tense the muscles by biting hard . . . Feel your jaw muscles
tighten . . . Feel the tension in your face . . . Across your forehead . . . Behind your eyes . . . In your jaw . . . Now let go . . .
Relax your forehead and drop your jaw . . . Feel the strain
easing . . . Feel the tension draining away from your face . . .
Your forehead feels smooth and relaxed . . . Your jaw is heavy
and loose . . . Imagine the tension leaving your face . . . Leaving
your neck . . . Draining away from your shoulders . . . Your
head, neck and shoulders feel heavy and relaxed. (REPEAT)
Think of your whole body now . . . Your entire body feels heavy and
relaxed . . . Let go of any tension . . . Imagine the tension flowing out of your body . . . Listen to the sound of your calm, even
breathing . . . Your arms, legs and head feel pleasantly heavy . . .
Too heavy to move . . . You may feel as though you are floating . . . Let it happen . . . It is part of being relaxed . . .
When images drift into your mind, don't fight them . . . Just
acknowledge them and let them pass . . . You are a bystander:*

interested but not involved . . . Enjoy the feelings of relaxation
for a few more moments . . . If you like, picture something that
gives you pleasure and a sense of calm . . .

In a moment, I will count backwards from four to one . . . When I
reach one, open your eyes and lie still for a little while before you
begin to move around again . . . You will feel pleasantly relaxed
and refreshed . . . Four: beginning to feel more alert . . . Three:
getting ready to start moving again . . . Two: aware of your
surroundings . . . One: eyes open, feeling relaxed and alert.

Shortened Relaxation Exercise

When the first exercise works for you, you can shorten the routine
by missing out the tensing stage. Alternatively, some people can
start the relaxation training at this stage because they already have
a good awareness of when they are tense and an ability to let it go.

INSTRUCTIONS:

You are relaxing . . . Breathe out slowly . . . Now, breathe in
smoothly and deeply . . . Now, breathe out slowly again, imagin-
ing yourself becoming heavier and heavier, sinking into the floor
(or your chair) . . . Keep breathing rhythmically, and feel a
sense of relief and of letting go . . . Try saying 'relax' to yourself
as you breathe out . . . Breathe like this for a few moments
more . . .

Now, begin to relax the muscles of your body . . . Think of your
feet . . . Let your feet go limp and floppy . . . Feel the tension
draining away from your feet . . . Let your feet roll outwards and
grow heavier and heavier . . . Imagine that they are so heavy
that they are sinking into the floor . . . More and more
relaxed . . . Growing heavier and more relaxed . . . (REPEAT)

Now, think about your calves . . . Let your feet touch the floor and
let your legs go floppy and heavy . . . Feel the tension leaving
your legs, draining away from your calves . . . Leaving your
calves feeling heavy . . . Draining away from your feet . . .
Leaving them feeling heavy and limp . . . Imagine that your legs

and feet are so heavy that they are sinking into the floor . . .
They feel limp and relaxed . . . Growing more and more heavy
and relaxed . . . (REPEAT)

Think about your thigh muscles . . . Feel the tension draining
away from your legs . . . They feel limp and heavy . . . Your
thighs feel heavy . . . Your calves feel heavy . . . Your feet feel
heavy . . . Imagine the tension draining away . . . Leaving your
legs . . . Leaving them feeling limp and relaxed . . . Leaving
them feeling so heavy that they are sinking into the floor (or
your chair) . . . Let the feelings of relaxation spread up from
your feet . . . Up through your legs . . . Relaxing your hips and
lower back . . . (REPEAT)

Now relax the muscles of your hips and lower back . . . If you feel
tension, let it go . . . Let your muscles relax . . . Feel your spine
supported . . . Feel the muscles relax . . . Deeper and deeper . . .
More and more relaxed . . . Growing heavier and heavier . . . Your
hips are relaxed . . . Your legs are relaxed . . . Your feet are
heavy . . . Tension is draining away from your body . . . (REPEAT)

Relax your stomach and chest muscles . . . As you breathe out, let go
of your tension . . . Feel your stomach muscles relax . . . Feel the
tightness leave your chest . . . As you breathe evenly and calmly,
your chest and stomach should gently rise and fall . . . Allow your
breathing to become rhythmic and relaxed . . . (REPEAT)

Now think about your hands and arms . . . Gently drop your arms
by your sides and imagine the tension draining away from your
arms . . . Leaving your upper arms . . . Leaving your fore-
arms . . . Draining away from your hands . . . Your arms feel
heavy and floppy . . . Your arms feel limp and relaxed . . .
(REPEAT)

Think about the muscles in your shoulders . . . Now relax . . . Let
your head drop forward . . . Let your shoulders drop . . . Let
them drop even further . . . Feel the tension easing away from
your neck and shoulders . . . Feel your muscles relaxing more
and more deeply . . . Your neck is limp, and your shoulders feel
heavy . . . (REPEAT)

Think about your face muscles . . . Focus on the muscles running across your forehead . . . Relax your forehead and drop your jaw . . . Feel the strain easing . . . Feel the tension draining away from your face . . . Your forehead feels smooth and relaxed . . . Your jaw is heavy and loose . . . Imagine the tension leaving your face . . . Leaving your neck . . . Draining away from your shoulders . . . Your head, neck and shoulders feel heavy and relaxed . . . (REPEAT)

Think of your whole body now . . . Your entire body feels heavy and relaxed . . . Let go of any tension . . . Imagine the tension flowing out of your body . . . Listen to the sound of your calm, even breathing . . . Your arms, legs and head feel pleasantly heavy . . . Too heavy to move . . . You may feel as though you are floating . . . Let it happen . . . It is part of being relaxed . . . When images drift into your mind, don't fight them . . . Just acknowledge them and let them pass . . . You are a bystander: interested but not involved . . . Enjoy the feelings of relaxation for a few more moments . . . If you like, picture something that gives you pleasure and a sense of calm . . .

In a moment, I will count backwards from four to one . . . When I reach one, open your eyes and lie still for a little while before you begin to move around again . . . You will feel pleasantly relaxed and refreshed . . . Four: beginning to feel more alert . . . Three: getting ready to start moving again . . . Two: aware of your surroundings . . . One: eyes open, feeling relaxed and alert.

Simple Relaxation Routine

Once deep relaxation has been mastered, or for those of you who might not need or want to use the longer exercises, you can introduce an even shorter exercise. This can be practised whenever it is needed. The following routine is based on a short exercise called Benson's 'Relaxation Routine' and it incorporates a mental image or sound into the relaxation exercise. This can be a pleasant, calming scene, such as a deserted beach; a particularly relaxing picture or object; a soothing sound or word, like the sound of the sea or the word 'serene'. The important thing is that you find something that is calming for you.

From time to time, distracting thoughts will come to mind – this is quite usual. Don't dwell on this; simply return to thinking about the soothing image or sound. Once you have started the exercise, and got into the rhythm of it, carry on for a minute or so. It's up to you to decide how much time you need to achieve a sense of relaxation.

INSTRUCTIONS:

To start the exercise, sit in a comfortable position. First, focus on your breathing. Take a slow, deep breath in . . . Feel the muscle beneath your ribcage move . . . Now let it out – slowly . . . Aim for a smooth pattern of breathing.

Close your eyes, and, while you continue to breathe slowly, imagine your body becoming more heavy . . . Scan your body for tension . . . Start at your feet and move up through your body to your shoulders and head . . . If you find any tension, try to relax that part of your body . . . Now, while your body is feeling as heavy and comfortable as possible, become aware of your breathing again . . . Breathe in through your nose, and fill your lungs fully . . . Now, breathe out again and bring to mind your tranquil image or sound . . . Breathe easily and naturally as you do this . . . Again, breathe in through your nose, filling your lungs, right down to your diaphragm . . . and out, thinking of your soothing picture or sound . . . When you are ready to breathe in again, repeat the cycle . . . Keep repeating this cycle until you feel relaxed and calm and refreshed . . .

When you have finished this exercise, sit quietly for a few moments, and enjoy the feeling of relaxation. Don't move around too quickly if you have been quite relaxed – take it gently.

All these exercises are a means to an end: the end point is you being able to recognise unproductive tension and respond by calming and relaxing yourself. Everyone will fare differently, and progress will have its ups and downs, so expect this and view setbacks as normal and as learning opportunities.

Distraction

A common response to upsetting thoughts and images is increased anxiety or lowered mood – which then fuels the problem cognitions and traps us in distressing cycles that can be really hard to break.

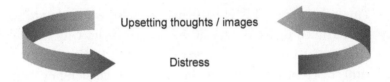

Upsetting thoughts / images

Distress

The very basic cognitive strategy of distraction rests on the idea that, although we can pay scant attention to several things at once, we can only really attend to one thing at a time. So, if we focus on something neutral or pleasant, we can avoid getting caught up with negative thoughts and urges: we can break out of these cycles.

Distraction can serve two purposes:

- Breaking unhelpful cycles of thoughts or images that might otherwise result in negative moods, increasing preoccupation and so on. This often offers immediate respite. Sometimes it is a temporary solution, giving a person time to recover and marshal their resources, but it sometimes actually results in problem management because of:
- Changing attitudes towards negative cognitions. Instead of getting caught up in them, distraction can help a person achieve distance from them and to see them as 'just thoughts' rather than convincing truths about themselves or the world.

Thinking about something positive is more effective than trying *not* to think about something negative. You can easily try this out for yourself – try *not* to think about pink balloons, for example, and your mind will probably fill with pink balloons and you won't be able to keep your mind free of them. If, on the other hand, your goal is to think about pink balloons and you try to do this, you will find that you succeed. Furthermore, you can probably manipulate the balloons in your imagination – you can make them rise or fall as you wish or have them explode, for example. This reminds us of the potential control that we have over images.

Distraction techniques include:

- *Physical exercise.* This is particularly useful when we are so preoccupied that it is very difficult to come up with mental challenges. Physical activities can be overt (e.g. going for a run), discreet (e.g. pelvic floor exercises), challenging (e.g. difficult yoga exercises) or mundane (e.g. household chores). The important thing is that they are engaging.
- *Refocusing.* This usually means paying attention to the external environment – and objects or people within it – rather than our internal world. Try describing to yourself what's around you – shapes, colours, smells, sounds, textures and so on. The more detailed the description, the more distracting the task will be. I've sat in many waiting rooms and ante-rooms in hospitals reading the notices on the walls (often backwards because this was more distracting) or counting the number of scuffs on the paintwork (this will usually keep a person very occupied in an NHS establishment) or following the sounds of hospital equipment to keep my mind off my worries when it was clear that worrying wasn't going to help me.
- *Mental exercise.* This simply means engaging our minds in mental exercises that might include tasks such as counting backwards in 7s from 100, or reciting a poem, or reconstructing in detail a favourite piece of music or scene from a movie. You might be able to make best use of this sort of mental distraction by carrying around a book or magazine that will grab your attention, or some photographs of loved ones or a special place, or by listening to music or talking books. Another

effective distraction is a self-created mental image of a place where you would like to be – a beach, a beautiful garden, a ski slope – whatever appeals to you. In order for this to be an effective distraction, the image should be attractive, filled with sensory details (smells, touch and sound as well as visual images), it should tell a story so that it keeps you engaged and most important of all it should be well-rehearsed so that it is easy to bring to mind even when you are stressed.

- *Counting cognitions.* Simply counting troubling thoughts or images can help us achieve a distance from them and this can break the distress cycle by dampening down the emotional impact of an upsetting cognition. This works because we stop paying attention to the *content* and simply count cognitions with the same attitude one might have to spotting how many pigeons there are in one's neighbourhood: 'There's one . . . and another . . . oh, and there's another!'

When using distraction exercises, remember to bear in mind:

- The exercise must suit you. For example, mental arithmetic and a beach image would not be effective for someone who hates mathematics and is allergic to sand. You'll only be able to engage in distraction if the exercise is readily accessible and attractive. Build on your interests and strengths.
- You might need several techniques to use under different circumstances. For example, tasks need to be discreet in a public place, whilst in private they can be more overt; physical strategies can be most accessible when we are highly preoccupied, and mental strategies more usable at lower levels of preoccupation. In the table below are a few of the things that helped me in the early days.
- Distraction will be counter-productive if we use it to avoid tackling things that need to be addressed or if we start to believe that we can't cope without it. Real problems do need to be tackled and we do need to build up (or rebuild)

self-confidence that we can cope so we should not become over-reliant on distraction. However, it can be a really helpful stepping stone at a time when we are struggling to cope.

- For some of us just breaking the cycle of worry or negative thinking can be enough to deal with unrealistic concerns but distraction does not fundamentally address persistent unhelpful thoughts or images, so it is not necessarily a good strategy for the long term: hence the need for the other strategies that CBT offers.

	At home	At work	In public
Low–moderate stress	Read my novel (keep it on my phone for easy access). Do physical work in the garden. Sing along to music (as long as I'm alone). Smelling soothing oils – vanilla-based ones work for me.	Prepare illustrations for teaching, trawling the internet for images. Review my calendar and my 'to-do' list. In a meeting: make notes of what's being said.	Try to remember the plot of the novel I'm reading and talk myself through it. Attend to the detail around me: smells, sounds, textures . . . On my phone, scroll through family pictures that are soothing and pleasurable. Listen to music through ear buds – try not to sing. Walk, keep moving.
High level stress	Go out for a walk if possible: make it brisk. Baking with the kids. Watch something easy and entertaining on TV or the internet – better still if this is with family.	Take a walk to the canteen, sometimes circling the hospital to get more exercise. Try to go with a colleague. Work through puzzles on my phone until I'm calm enough to do something more productive. In a meeting: doodle until I'm calm enough to start taking notes again.	Mentally describe in detail what I can see: whatever is in shop windows / the number of red cars or people carrying handbags, etc. In waiting areas, use puzzles, the news pages, etc., on my phone. Count down from 100 in multiples of 7.

Templates

Thought Diary

You can use a grid like the one on the next page to catch the thoughts or images that trigger distress. It is a pretty basic grid and you can add to it in all sorts of useful ways if and when the time is right for you.

For example, some people find it helpful to:

- **Note the time and date** – this can help us recognise patterns to feeling distressed and if we can identify patterns we can predict what will upset us and sometimes it's possible to anticipate and prepare for the difficult times.
- **State what the distress feels like** – misery, fear, anger, for example. In this way you can begin to get a better idea of what thoughts or images link with what emotions and some-times this better understanding of distress can help us better manage our emotions.
- **Use a distress rating** – maybe using a 5-point scale where 1 represents no distress and 5 means as distressed as possible. If you rate your distress when you first have the thought or image and later when you have reviewed it, you can see how well the technique is working for you. We would hope that the distress rating would fall over time – however, don't be disheartened if this doesn't happen immediately. It is common to experience a bit of a 'head-heart gap': a delay between what your head knows and what your heart feels.
- **Use a belief rating** – some people find it helpful to rate how strongly they believe their initial distressing thought and how strongly they believe their newly reviewed thought, a thought that we hope is more soothing or assuring. Again, a simple 1–5 rating scale might be sufficient and again this is a way of seeing how well the technique works for you. When the technique is working you will see a steady rise in your belief rating of your new, more positive perspective.

These are all options – you don't have to make the thought diary complicated; you simply need to make it work for you. Some people will get the most out of a template that collects more information while others will find that the simple grid is best for them. Experiment and see.

Thought / Image (Optional rating)	It's no wonder I think this . . .	. . . on the other hand . . .	Rethink the thought (Optional rating)

Activity Grid

The activity grid on page 170 is the simplest of templates and you can adapt it however you need to in order to get the best use out of it.

Sometimes you might merge some of the cells because you do the same thing for several hours – sleeping or watching TV, for example. Sometimes you might need to split a cell because you spend time on more than one activity in an hour. Personalise the grid so that it captures the information that you need, don't try to force your day into the boxes.

When I used the grid, I added ratings out of 10 (where 1 was low and 10 was high) for:

- **Pleasure (P)**: noting how much enjoyment certain activities gave me and then I'd try to build on this and incorporate as much 'P' as possible.
- **Purposefulness/Satisfaction (PS)**: noting how useful and meaningful an activity was. Again, I'd try to then incorporate as many 'PS' activities as I could when I planned ahead.

Some people like to use a rating that indicates how difficult a task is and therefore what an achievement it is to have carried it out:

- **Difficulty/Achievement (DA)**: this enables us to give ourselves credit for doing the things that are hard right now. For some of us this is simply getting out of bed or carrying out daily chores. By recognising how difficult an activity is we are acknowledging the effort it demands. Then we can take credit for trying or we can be compassionate if we found it too hard.

The grids can be used in two ways. Initially they are useful in collecting information about our activities so that we can see what we find pleasurable, satisfying and difficult. Later we can build on this by using the grid to plan the days or week ahead, maximising the things that make us feel better and more satisfied.

	Monday	Tuesday	Wednesday	Thursday	Friday	Saturday	Sunday
6.00–7.00							
7.00–8.00							
8.00–9.00							
9.00–10.00							
10.00–11.00							
11.00–12.00							
12.00–1.00							
1.00–2.00							
2.00–3.00							
3.00–4.00							
4.00–5.00							
5.00–6.00							
6.00–7.00							
7.00–8.00							
8.00–9.00							
9.00–11.00							

Acknowledgements

Where to start? So very many people showed kindness and under-standing from the moment that the ambulance crew arrived and gently and competently set Udo on the long road to recovery. En route we have been grateful to the professionals who absolutely lived up to the friends and family who ensured that we were supported and even fed. Udo's former patients and colleagues sent warm wishes that buoyed him up in the bleakest times, and the book contract from the team at Robinson at Little, Brown Book Group gave him purpose when he felt most adrift.

But, without wishing to sink into Oscar-ceremony sentimental-ity, our greatest appreciation is reserved for our daughter and son. Alongside us they experienced trauma, loss and relentless stress, and yet they never complained and they didn't demand. In fact, they brought cheer into our strange new lives and they were the best incentive for soldiering on. They reminded us that, despite everything, there is good reason to feel blessed.

Index

Page numbers in *italics* refer to images